CRYSTAL ENCHANTMENTS

A Complete Guide to Stones and Their Magical Properties

D. J. Conway

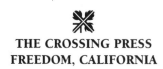

THE CROSSING PRESS
FREEDOM, CALIFORNIA

For information on bulk purchases or group discounts for this and other Crossing Press titles, please contact our Special Sales Manager at 800/777-1048.
Visit our Web site: **www.crossingpress.com**

Cautionary Note: The information contained within this book is in no way intended as a substitute for medical counseling. Please do not attempt self-treatment of a medical problem without consulting a qualified health practitioner.

The author and The Crossing Press expressly disclaim any and all liability for any claims, damages, losses, judgements, expenses, costs, and liabilities of any kind or injuries resulting from any products offered in this book by participating companies and their employees or agents. Nor does the inclusion of any resource group or company listed within this book constitute an endorsement or guarantee of quality by the author or The Crossing Press.

Library of Congress Cataloging-in-Publication Data

Conway, D.J. (Deanna J.)
    Crystal enchantments / by D.J. Conway.
        p. cm.
    Includes bibliographical references and index.
    ISBN 1-58091-010-6 (pbk.)
        1. Crystals--Psychic aspects.. 2. Precious stones--Psychic aspects.
    3. Magic. I. Title.
    BF1442.P74C66 2000
    133'.2548--dc211   99-36233
                                                             CIP

Contents

Part I

GATE OF STONE

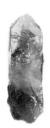

The Magical Allure of Stones

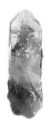

It is not unusual anymore to see people wearing rock crystal or amethyst points hung on chains and earrings, or set in rings. Geodes, crystal clusters, crystal balls, or solitary crystals decorate office desks, homes, or little altars. Set small children down with a box of tumbled stones, and they will entertain themselves for quite some time. Even adults find it a satisfying, relaxing pastime. Many people consider this attraction to crystals and other stones a modern era, New Age phenomenon, but this is hardly the case. The magical allure of stones has attracted humans for thousands of years.

From the very earliest times, humans have been intrigued by and drawn to stones. Not only did these early humans use various stones to make tools and weapons, but they sensed the magic within certain stones and learned to use that as well. Stones became the gateway to the use of psychic powers, healing, spiritual development, protection, and divine guidance. We commonly think of the ancient Egyptians when we think of the ancient uses of stones. However, the stone history goes back much further than that.

Archaeologists have determined from their excavation discoveries that the people of the Upper Paleolithic Period (25,000–12,000 B.C.E.) were already decorating themselves with shells, pieces of bone, teeth, and unique pebbles. One of the most sacred stones in this period was amber.

Cultures in Mesopotamia in the seventh millennium B.C.E. fashioned beads of carnelian and rock crystal. About 2,000 years later, in the same region, they were engraving cylinder seals of such stones as steatite and marble; by the fourth millennium they also made seals of rock crystal.

The ancient Indus civilization of the third millennium B.C.E. was working with a great many gemstones available in that region of India. A woman's belt, recovered during excavations in Harappa, clearly represents the gemstones known and used by this culture: red carnelian, green steatite, agate, jasper, amazonite, jade, and lapis lazuli. Very early works in Sanskrit on astrology (400 B.C.E.) detail the power of the known stones of that region.

Lapis lazuli mines were operating in Afghanistan about 5000 years ago, as were turquoise mines on the Sinai Peninsula. Evidence of a thriving export trade in gems has been found throughout the Mediterranean area and, in some cases, well beyond this. Afghanistan lapis was reaching Egypt well before 3000 BCE and ancient Sumer by 2500 B.C.E.. Gems from the same mining sources have been traced to Greece, Rome, India, and even China.

The Phoenicians, who were great travelers and sea merchants, traded for amber around the Baltic Sea, then carried it for sale to North Africa, Turkey, Cyprus, and Greece. This has been confirmed by spectroscopic analysis of amber beads found in graves of Mycenaean Greece.[1] Amber beads found in Crete and England have been dated from 2000 B.C.E., while amber pendants and beads discovered in Estonia date from 3,700 B.C.E.. After the time of Alexander the Great (356–323 BCE), trade between the East and West increased, thus bringing many new gemstones to light.

Our greatest knowledge of the Egyptian use of gemstones comes from tomb excavations, particularly that of Tutankhamen, who reigned from 1361 to 1352 B.C.E.. The Egyptians' strong belief in an afterlife caused them to use many stones to protect the dead and bring them good luck with the Underworld judges. Archaeologists found 143 pieces of jewelry with the mummy of Tutankhamen; these were made of gold, carnelian, jasper, lapis lazuli, turquoise, obsidian, rock crystal, alabaster, amazonite, and jade. In contrast to the Babylonians who were not too concerned about an afterlife, the Egyptian jewels often show little everyday wear.

Gemstones set in rings were a late addition to human adornment. Rings made of gold, silver, iron, carved amber, and ivory were the first types worn by the Egyptians, Greeks, Etruscans, and other Mid-Eastern cultures. These rings were plain in the beginning, then gradually became signet rings, used in the same way as the cylinder seals for signing documents. Bronze Age rings from a Scythian settlement on the Caspian Sea have been dated to the second millennium BCE. There is a clay tablet from the reign of Artaxerxes I of Persia that records the sale of a gold and emerald ring. In fact, this tablet contains a guarantee that the stones will not fall out for twenty years, something you could not possibly get a dealer to sign today.

When gemstones began to be set in rings (a different date for each culture), setting stones in necklaces, earrings, bracelets, pins, and hair ornaments quickly followed. By the time of Imperial Rome, it was common to give birthday rings (*anuli natalitii*).

The later Greeks began to collect information and write about the medicinal qualities of gemstones. These mineralogical and medical texts were called lapidaries. Many of the virtues and astrological symbolism connected with stones in these writings come from earlier Arabic lapidaries. The oldest surviving mineralogy book, *On Stones*, was written by the Greek Theophratus (c. 372–287 B.C.E.), who was considered to be the successor of Aristotle. Another early Greek lapidary was written by Damigeron; this was later translated into Latin between the first and sixth centuries. The 37-volume *Historia Naturalis* was written by Pliny the Elder (23–79 C.E.), who compiled all the information of his predecessors; however, only volume 37 had anything on precious stones. Pliny was killed while watching the eruption of Mt. Vesuvius.

By the eighth century, similar European texts began to appear, as well as one by the Arab Avicenna (980–1073). In the eleventh century, Marbode, bishop of Rennes, produced a rather elaborate text on stones. In thirteenth century Germany, *Steinbuch* by Volmar was printed, along with *De Mineralibus* by Albertus Magnus (1206–1280). *De Natura Fossilium*, a text on stones and their physical properties, was written by Georgius Agricola in 1546 and *De Re Metallica*, a book on mining, in 1556.[2]

Medieval Europeans believed in wearing medicinal amulets made of certain stones or taking the virtues of these stones as a potion. Of course, only the wealthy could afford this practice. Their interest in the subject spawned the compilation of even more books on the subject: *Speculum Lapidum* by Camillus Leonardus of Venice in 1502; *de Gemmis et Coloribus* by Geronimo Cardano in 1587; *Gemmarum et Lapidum Historia* by Anselmus Boetius de Boot in 1609.

Travel books by Marco Polo in the thirteenth century and Jean Baptiste Tavernier in the seventeenth century also held valuable information on gems, their uses, and sources.

Although certain gems have gone in and out of favor over the centuries, gemstones have never lost their allure. In the beginning, the magic of stones was within the reach of any person who could find the kind she/he wanted. Then stones and their powers became the province of the wealthy. Now, once again, everyone has the opportunity to own stones and use their magic. All it takes is common sense, practice, patience, and determination.

The gate of stone is the gateway to spiritual and psychic advancement through the correct use of stones and gems. Stones and gems are tools that aid in our search for betterment of our lives on all levels. I have compiled this book to help those who search for another meaningful way to improve themselves. Although intentional stone magic, as opposed to merely collecting stones, is serious magic, it should also be approached with a sense of fun and anticipation. A day when something new is learned is a day not wasted. Even if you should never attempt the magical procedures, you can gain from just learning about and handling stones. Hopefully, this book will help you to open the gate of stone and pass through into the land of gem enchantment.

Preparing for Stone Magic

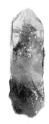

Many people start their relationship with stones as children. They pick up and take home little colored stones encountered along the road or on the beach during a walk. Not every stone will do, however. Only certain ones are given the honor of being placed in the "treasure box" in the bottom drawer. Size, color, and shape have no bearing. If you were to ask a child why she/he choose the one in her/his hand and not the one left on the ground, the child would have difficulty explaining, except "I like the way it feels."

As adults wanting to renew our relationship with stones, we need to regain the child's skill of disregarding looks and choosing the ones that silently call to us, that feel good. This is not difficult with a little practice.

Everyone has one hand that is stronger in sensing and sending power than the other. Usually this power hand is the one you basically use the most and with which you write. However, there are a few people whose power hand is the one they use least in daily life; this does not happen often, but can occur. Also, there are people whose power hand will change from one hand to the other, although they probably will not change their writing hand.

The power hand is used to sense a stone's vibrations and its compatibility of vibrations with yours. When choosing a stone, whether from Nature or in a rock shop, pick up the first one that attracts your eyes. Hold the stone loosely in your power hand. It may feel hot, cold, or anything in between. It may feel "sharp," "comforting," "vibrating," or "slimy." The important thing is how you feel about it when holding it. Sometimes, closing your eyes helps to sense the stone's vibrations better, especially in the beginning of your work with stones. If you do not feel comfortable with that particular stone, don't buy it, regardless of how much you want it or how low the price is. It does not match your vibrations and will often only bring you difficulties. If the stone has a very negative, or slimy, feeling, don't take it, even if it is offered to you as a gift. These types of vibrations will draw more of the same into your life.

After obtaining a stone or stones, cleanse them as soon as you get home. Then spend time each day getting acquainted with them. Hold them, look at them, feel all their shapes and angles. Press each one lightly against the center of your forehead between your eyes. Watch for mental flashes of color, brief pictures, sounds, and feelings. Get to know each of your stones before using it in any magical spells.

There are several ways to cleanse unwanted vibrations from stones. If the stone is mounted in jewelry, you can hold it in cool, running water for several minutes; then carefully dry it. Cold water is not advisable on such stones as opals and turquoise, because they react negatively to sudden temperature changes and may shatter. Follow this by holding the stone in the smoke of frankincense, myrrh, or lotus incense. Then quickly wave it through the heat at the top of the flame of a burning candle.

If the stone is unset, and not one of the fragile types, you can bury it in a small bowl of salt for a time. This time period can range from one hour to two days, depending upon how the stone feels when you take it out of the salt. Then rinse it thoroughly under cool, running water and dry. Salt is not advisable on certain stones, such as pearls, opals, or turquoise. Also, dispose of the salt when finished, as it is now contaminated with possible negative vibrations and should not be used again.

Another method is to soak the stone in a mixture of one-half cup salt to one quart of cool water for several hours, again depending upon how much the stone needs to be cleansed. If the stone is particularly dirty in a physical sense, you can use an old toothbrush to gently remove bits of debris.

If you want something different from the salt methods, you can bury the stone in earth for three days. Apartment dwellers need not despair; you can use fresh potting soil in a flowerpot for this. Then hold it under cool water, in incense smoke, and candle heat.

Whichever method you use, it is always wise to follow the primary cleansing method by holding the stone in incense smoke and waving it above the flame of a candle. This seems to seal the cleaned stone and allows it to build up its power faster.

If you are attempting to clean soft stones, such as calcite, you never want to put them in any water. Instead, use incense smoke and candle heat as a cleanser. Water will destroy soft stones.

Now you have your stones, or at least a few of them. Some stones you will want to display, but others you will want to store for magical use. These are the stones you really do not want other people handling indiscriminately. Since it is often easy to forget which stone is which, you can keep each stone in a separate little box or plastic bag with the name written on it. Set aside a drawer to house your stones. Or you can purchase one of the small plastic boxes with drawers that are available for jewelry or lingerie. If the drawers do not have dividers, make your own out of strips of cardboard. Label each section so you can identify the stone in it.

Before you begin to use your stones, read up on each one in the following section. You will be amazed at the history behind a great many of the world's gemstones. Mineralogy is a fascinating study. So is the historical use of stones in magic and healing, although mineralogists tend to look down their noses at these meanings. Decide for yourself through practice and hands-on use.

As with any magic, you need to be responsible for the stone magic you do. Rather than doing a spell to make a certain person love you, for example, work the magic to bring you your perfect love. Likewise, do not perform magic to control or harm another person. Negative magic of any kind will eventually bring home to you unpleasant results that will only complicate your life further. The whole idea behind magic is to make your life, your surroundings, and the world better, not worse.

A good many celebrities believe in the powers of stones and carry or wear them often, if not all the time. Demi Moore wears a special protection crystal around her neck, as does Patrick Swayze. Both Cybill Shepherd and Michael York carry a selection of different stones. Other believers in the powers of stones include Liz Taylor, Oprah Winfrey, Boy George, Wynonna Judd, John Travolta, and Johnny Carson. So if you like to have stone power around you, you are in good company.

Keep an open mind when learning to use the power of stones. A closed mind with preconceived ideas never accomplishes much, nor does it recognize the unexpected wonders that come its way. You need an open mind to go through the gate of stone and expand your magical knowledge.

Part II

STONES AND THEIR POWERS

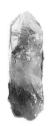

A Few Facts

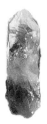

Minerals are chemicals that were blended during the Earth's formation to produce a distinct set of characteristics. Each mineral has a "fingerprint," or make-up, which makes it distinguishable from other minerals. Quartz, for example, is the most common mineral in the Earth's crust. Although there are thousands of different minerals, only about fifty of them are known and used as gemstones in jewelry. A number of the remainder are cut only for collections, as they are too soft to be worn in jewelry.

Gemstones are classified in several different ways, one of which is hardness. This list, called the Moh's scale, runs from diamond, which is a 10 and the hardest gemstone we know, down to talc, which is a 1 and is extremely soft. Of the five major gemstones—diamond, ruby, sapphire, emerald, and pearl—the first three are at or near the top of the list in hardness. A very few gems, such as kyanite, have a different hardness across their width than they do along their length.

The commonly listed twelve top gemstones are diamond, ruby, sapphire, emerald, aquamarine, chrysoberyl, topaz, tourmaline, peridot, garnet, pearl, and opal. This list may change at any time according to popularity, which is determined by current tastes and scarcity.

All inorganic gemstones are measured in carat weight. Carat is a standard weight worldwide; one carat equals 0.2 grams; the accepted international carat weight is 200 milligrams. The word carat originated in the Middle East, where once gems were weighed against carob seeds. The Arabic word for the carob seed is *quirat*. This seed is a product of the carob tree and has a fairly consistent weight. Faceted gems are measured in points; one hundred points equals one carat of gem.

The word karat is the measurement of gold purity and does not apply to gems. If gold is twenty-five karats, it is pure, with no other metals present. However, pure gold has only a hardness of 2.5, which is far too soft for jewelry. Therefore, other metal alloys are added to give it strength.

Organic gemstones are also considered valuable because they are beautiful, scarce, and unusual. Sometimes these stones are produced by creatures, as with pearl, coral, shell, and ivory. Other times they are formed by natural Earth processes over thousands of years, as with amber, jet, fossils, and petrified wood.

Some of the magical uses of stones that I give will differ from the uses listed by other writers. These are based on my personal experiences with stones. However, the traditional uses are given as well as my own. Some stones are so "new" to humans that these stones have no magical traditions or uses associated with them. By "new" I mean that they are not listed in old texts, have been renamed and separated from stones with which they were previously connected, or have been recently discovered. It will be up to individual magicians to experiment with them to discover the best magical uses, beyond those I list.

It is not necessary to buy a large, expensive stone in order to work magic with it. A small piece that is not gem quality can work just as well as a large piece. As with any stone, you should check the feel of each stone before you purchase it. Neither is it necessary to buy faceted or set stones. Natural and tumbled stones ordinarily have as much power as those that have been polished and cut, sometimes even more.

Manmade synthetic stones are often sneered at by magicians as being inferior in comparison to the natural, mined stones. However, most often this is unjustified. Good-quality synthetic stones are fully crystalline and differ only marginally from the natural stones, although they will have different inclusions from the mined stones. Synthetic stones also will have the same refraction, physical and optical qualities, and chemical composition as the real thing. It is often difficult for even a gem expert to tell the difference between a natural and a synthetic stone without the use of a microscope and special tests. When purchasing a synthetic stone, be certain that it is a genuine synthetic and not a simulated or artificial stone.

The manufacture of synthetic stones is a fairly recent process in the history of gems. Simulated and artificial stones only marginally look like the real gem and are not anywhere near the same in physical properties. Artificial stones are deliberately made of glass or polystyrene latex to imitate more expensive gems, while simulated stones are actual stones made to look like other more expensive ones. Simulated stones are changed by heating, staining, oils, and irradiation. Artificial and simulated stones have been manufactured for centuries to fool both the buyer and friends of a purchaser who wish others to think they own the real gems.

Sometimes expensive stones are simulated (and the cost to the gem seller cut) by cementing a thin section of the natural stone on top of a colored glass base; called a doublet, this faked stone gives the appearance of a large, genuine gem except for the tiny junction point between the thin slab of gem and the glass base. Sometimes a triplet (three layers) is made, particularly with artificial opals, with a top dome of rock crystal, a very thin middle layer of precious opal, and a base of glass, potch (common) opal, or chalcedony. This type of "simulated" stone can still be valuable for magical work as a genuine piece of the authentic stone is there.

To begin working magic with stones, choose the least expensive ones. Store each in a box or a small plastic bag with a closure top and put a label with the name of the stone on the container. Store all your magical stones in a special box or drawer; this keeps them from picking up unwanted vibrations from other people or the atmosphere in the house. Handle your stones frequently, and learn to appreciate their long history. If you have a stone set in jewelry, you can still use it in magical spellworkings. I found, more times than not, that the silver or gold mounting enhanced the magic instead of detracted from it.

Some of the stones in the following list are not actually inorganic stones, but beautiful, Nature-created organic materials that have been used in jewelry and magic for centuries. Their powers and allure earn them the right to be among your magical equipment.

Amulets and talismans are often spoken of in the use of magic.

These words are not interchangeable as they have two different and distinct meanings. An amulet is a specific stone or medallion that, because of the virtues in its very being, protects the wearer. The name probably comes from either the Arabic word *hamalat* ("something worn") or the Latin word *amuletum,* which comes from the verb *amoliri* ("drive away"). A talisman is a specific stone or medallion that is spelled to bring something to the wearer or user. The word talisman probably originated with the Arabic word *tilsam,* which found its way into the Greek language, where it was defined as "an initiation or incantation."

The oldest magic formulas still preserved were written down by the Sumerians; some of these contain references to stone magic and amulets. They also refer to two stones which the Sumerians and Assyrians considered very important: the aban rame ("stone of love") and the aban la rame ("stone of non-love").[1] We have no clues to what actual stones these were as there are no descriptions. Until well into the seventeenth century, princes and peasants alike in Europe, the Middle East, and the Far East believed in and used the magical virtues of stones, wearing them as amulets and talismans.

The Eastern countries, such as India, have long used specific stones to remedy or counteract the negative effect of malefic planets in astrological charts. The earliest Sanskrit work on the subject, the *Vishnu-Purana,* is dated to about the second century B.C.E. In one list, ruby was worn to correct an ill-aspected Sun, cat's-eye for the Moon, coral for Mars, yellow sapphire for Mercury, pearl for Jupiter, diamond for Venus, blue sapphire for Saturn, onyx for the North Node of the Moon, and emerald for the South Node. Another list gives pearl for the Moon, emerald for Mercury, yellow sapphire for Jupiter, and cat's-eye for the South Node.

Although stone aids for health are listed, do not substitute these for a medical doctor's care and advice. Instead, use the power of the appropriate stones as an additional aid to standard treatment.

The following chapters describe stones, their hardness, color, source, and healing and magical uses.

Adularia

▶ **HARDNESS:** 6

▶ **COLORS:** Colorless or pale gray, sometimes with a blue, silvery white, or white schiller (sheen).

▶ **SOURCES:** Switzerland, Sri Lanka, Madagascar, Myanmar, Burma, Australia, India, Tanzania, Brazil, and the U.S.

▶ **FACTS:** A member of the orthoclase (an alkali feldspar) family, adularia is a kind of moonstone. Orthoclase gets its name from the Greek for "break straight." This refers to the stone's perfect cleavage. The adularia found in Switzerland has a bluish sheen, and the stone takes its name from the Adular-Bergstock area of that country.

This type of moonstone has a turbid transparency that is softer and more diffuse than the other chatoyant stones. Cleavage cracks may be visible inside the stone. Its value is fairly low; however, the stones that exhibit a blue reflection are highly prized.

▶ **HISTORY AND FOLKLORE:** Adularia moonstone has the same historical background as feldspar moonstone. Neither stone is selenite, which is a form of gypsum, soft and very fragile.

This stone is connected with the Moon and the signs of Cancer, Libra, and Scorpio.

To dream of adularia means the revealing of secrets.

▶ **HEALING ENERGIES:** This stone can be calming to the nerves. Healers use it to treat ulcers, edema, and emotional problems. See Moonstone.

▶ **MAGICAL POWERS:** Adularia is a visionary stone, like feldspar moonstone. Helps one to see all the possibilities in any situation. Aids in defining all positives and negatives in planning a goal or desire. See Moonstone.

MAGICAL USES

Most of the available adularia is not of the beautifully clear gem quality we see in feldspar moonstone. However, this does not preclude its use in magical undertakings. Tuck a piece or several pieces in the drawer or box that holds your favorite divination tools. Before laying out cards or casting the runes, hold the piece of adularia in both hands and bring it up to your third eye in the center of your forehead. Silently ask for direction and guidance. Then lay the stone near the center of the area where you will be placing your cards or runes. This opens your psychic intuition and aids in giving a correct and helpful reading. Other uses are the same as listed under Moonstone.

Agate

▶ **HARDNESS:** 7

▶ **COLOR:** There are many varieties and colors of agate.

▶ **SOURCES:** Found around the world. Huge quantities of agate are imported from such South American countries as Brazil and Paraguay. Good-quality agate also comes from the Deccan Valley of India. Idar-Oberstein in Germany is famous for its agate.

▶ **FACTS:** All agate is a type of quartz known as chalcedony. Its crypto-crystalline fibers can only be seen under a microscope. Agate is distinguished from other forms of chalcedony by its banded patterns, which are especially visible when the agate is cut and polished. Bands of various colors were formed around one or more centers by minerals deposited in ancient lava cavities, thus producing the agate. Agate with straight layers or bands is called ribbon agate; when the bands are in a zigzag formation, it is known as fortification agate.

The agate is a very porous stone that readily accepts chemicals. Because of the agate's ability to change color through chemicals and heating, there are whole industries devoted to producing chemically colored stones.

▶ **HISTORY AND FOLKLORE:** According to the Greek writer Theophrastus (c. 370–285 B.C.E.), the agate got its name from the River Achates on the island of Sicily, where the stone was found in large quantities. Today the River Achates is known as the River Dirillo.

A remaining fragment of a Greek work on amulets, written in the third or fourth century C.E., mentions an amulet set with the *ophiokiolus* stone, which protects sailors and travelers against the surging ocean. Since this stone is described as being girded with stripes like a snake, it was probably a banded agate.

In Rome, the reddish yellow agate, known as lion agate, was prized by the gladiators, not only for victory, but also for attracting the love of women.

Followers of Islam engraved agate with the symbols of the Prophet's grandsons and hung the stones about the necks of children to prevent falls and accidents. Many religious followers of Islam use necklaces made of various colors of agate. Ancient Jewish folklore also states that the agate protects against stumbling and falling. This belief was held for centuries by horsemen, who wove agate into the manes of horses and set it into the harnesses. It is very probable that this belief for protection of animals got changed when it reached Europe where farmers tied agates to the horns of oxen or the harness of horses when plowing fields; it was said to promote fertility of the crops.

In the 1500s in Italy the agate was said to turn away lightning and the destructive power of storms.

In certain parts of England, farmers still take an agate with a naturally bored hole through it and hang it on a nail over the door to the barn or stable. This is said to stop evil spirits from riding the cows and horses at night, and keep thunder and lightning from souring the milk.

The Vikings and people of Saxon England used a double-headed ax and a round agate to find lost articles or buried treasure. They did this by performing a magical divination known as axino-mancia. They heated the ax head until it glowed red, then pushed the handle into the ground so it stood upright. The round agate was then placed on the red-hot head. If the agate fell off, they were to look in the direction the stone rolled. If it stuck, what they sought was far away. A tenth century Anglo-Saxon manuscript also recommends agate as a defense against the devil and the assaults he might provoke through human allies.

The Book of Saxon Leechdoms, written in 1864, states that agate can protect not only from storms, sorcery, demonic possession, disease, poison, and drunkenness, but also from skin eruptions.

While the people in western Africa prefer green, white, and red agates, only the white agate is considered to give positive effects in northern Africa. In Ghana, agate amulets are worn or carried against snake bite, paralysis, and mental illness.

Wearing or carrying agate was said to prevent seasickness, while wearing it in a ring or pendant brought deep sleep, calmness, good health, long life, and sweetened the disposition.

The ancient writer Dioscorides, in his fifth book of the *Materia Medica* series, tells of over two hundred stones, among them agate, used for medicinal purposes by Roman physicians. A mixture of powdered agate and sweet fruit juice was given for insanity, ulcers, boils, and diseases of the kidneys and spleen. Certain types of agates were used to stop hemorrhages and combat epidemics and plagues. Worn as pendants, agates were recommended for indigestion, lung problems, and irrational fears. Arab physicians warned against taking powdered agate internally but used it in a paste to stop gum bleeding.

Red agate (also known as blood agate) was said to protect against spiders and scorpions. Green agate was highly prized and thought to be potent against any eye disease; in Syria women drank the water poured over a green agate to avoid sterility. In Egypt, gray agate was worn to prevent stiff neck and repel diarrhea and other intestinal problems; in Syria, triangularly-cut agates were worn for the same reasons. Although black agate with white stripes was highly prized, it was not considered as valuable as brown or tawny agate. Brown agate was said to be the most powerful of the agates, giving victory to the warrior, protecting from all poisonous reptiles, healing the sick, increasing the intelligence, repelling fevers and madness, and attracting love, riches, happiness, and long life.

In ancient Britain, agate was worn to prevent falls and to guard against skin diseases. In the Middle East, agate was believed to purify the blood. Red veins in agate were said to be the solidified blood of the gods.

Ordinary agate is often associated with Mercury and the signs Virgo and Gemini.

Dreaming of banded agate means a voyage on water. To dream of agate in general signifies a journey.

▶ **HEALING ENERGIES:** Wear to cure insomnia and give pleasant dreams. All agate can reverse the energy flow in any chakra, thus removing blockages and illnesses.

Tawny: held in the hand, it speeds recovery from illnesses.

▶ **MAGICAL POWERS:** Grounding but energetic, the agate can be used to strengthen the mind and body, give courage, ferret out the truth, or heal. Guards against all dangers; averts lightning and storms; gives strength and victory in endeavors; opens the wearer to receive unexpected favors from the deities. If used in sacred rituals as a divine object, it turns the words of your enemies against themselves. Agate increases balance on all levels. It is also useful when sudden bursts of energy, physical or mental, are needed.

Use in protective spells to guard against black magic, troublesome spirits, and negative thoughtforms. In Asia polished agate was used for scrying.

Black: prosperity, victory for athletes, courage.

Black with white stripes: creates alertness.

Blue with white stripes: visionary, psychic, dreams.

Brecchiated (broken agate pieces, usually brown, held together by quartz): optimism, tranquility, helps to avoid negative behavior; vibrational changer.

Brown: victory in conflicts; increases intelligence.

Creamy yellow: helps to lighten moods.

Enhydritic (nodules with water trapped inside): contact water devas; balance emotions.

Gray with white stripes: intellectual pursuits.

Leopard (pale yellow, brown or pink with leopard-like spots): called wolfstone at one time; excellent for taking back your personal power.

Lilac with pale blue gray stripes: spiritual discrimination.

Mustard yellow: useful in contacting the creative side of the mind and building an inventive mood.

Orange and brown: a balancer that aids in overcoming obstacles, gaining good luck in monetary issues, and stabilizing the emotions.

Pale blue with white lacy patterns: gives sense of security and ability to handle new situations; softens stubbornness.

Purple with threads of white: helps communications be powerful and to the point.

Red: peace, calmness; also said to drive away spiders.

Turquoise with white pattern (found in Hawaii): meet and make new friends.

MAGICAL USES

Carry slices of agate and handle them frequently to relieve stress or gain whatever power that color and variety exudes. This works in much the same manner as the worry stones of the Eastern cultures.

Sometimes you are fortunate enough to find a piece of sliced agate that is dark or black agate around the rim and with a center of crystal that has grown in a fractured pattern. These stones are especially valuable to those wishing to develop and strengthen the psychic ability of farseeing. The compelling design within the center section of crystal will not reveal itself until held up toward the light or with a candle flame behind it. Gaze at the lighted center, letting your mind open and gently drift. Symbols, patterns, and images will soon appear briefly, so you must be alert at the same time. Each time you view this center the images will be different. Also listen for mental messages from the astral to help you interpret what you see.

Eye Agate

▶ **COLORS:** Certain brown and black agates with a circular layer of a lighter color, often red or white.

▶ **FACTS:** These agates can be cut and polished to show an oval or round outline, resembling an eye.

▶ **HISTORY AND FOLKLORE:** Known as agate eye stones, these were highly prized in northern Africa and throughout the Mediterranean area and the Middle East as a talisman against the evil eye or ill-wishing. At one time in the city of Alleppo in Syria, these eye stones were used in the belief that they could heal a certain type of boil that looked very much like the eye of the stone.

A remaining fragment of the Greek work on amulets, mentioned earlier, also describes an amulet set with the *druops* stone, which was used against the evil eye. The *druops* is described as being white in the center, a description of an eye agate.

Eye agate has long been considered as excellent a scrying device as a quartz crystal ball. It symbolizes the third eye in the center of the forehead and is associated with the pineal gland.

Eye agate is associated with the Goddess and the sign of Virgo.

To dream of eye agate is a warning to keep alert; something unexpected will be happening.

▶ **HEALING ENERGIES:** Relieves tired eyes.

▶ **MAGICAL POWERS:** All eye agates turn aside ill-wishing from others. They also symbolize the protection of one's guardian spirit. Scrying, as with a crystal ball.

MAGICAL USES

If you experience troubled sleep and/or nightmares, put a piece of eye agate under your pillow at night. This will return any negative thoughtforms to the senders. Often you will be given valuable information during dreams; information that can help you to gain control of your life and sever any controlling cords (astral energy lines) from other people.

Spheres of eye agate can also be used as scrying devices.

Fire Agate

▶ **COLOR:** Usually a brownish color, with the fire bubbles visible only after careful cutting and polishing.

▶ **SOURCES:** Mexico and the southwestern U.S. This stone is a mineral of arid regions.

▶ **FACTS:** The fire agate is a fascinating stone of iridescent colors, sometimes called the iris agate and mud opal. Its flame-like colors, brought out by cutting *en cabochon*, are caused by thin layers of iron oxide crystals inside the stone. These iron oxide inclusions

give the stone an oily, fiery look, but only when the stone is polished. The background is a rather rusty brown.

Fire agate is entirely different from the Mexican fire opal,
although some jewelers will try to tell you they are the same.

▶ **HISTORY AND FOLKLORE:** Fire agate is associated with Mars and the
sign of Aries.

To dream of fire agate symbolizes emotionally upsetting experiences that can be dealt with positively if you keep your head.

▶ **HEALING ENERGIES:** Because of its grounding ability, this stone can
help take the edge off difficult emotionally charged problems.

▶ **MAGICAL POWERS:** Increases personal power and the ability to
operate efficiently where action is needed. Creates a good eye for
strategy. Useful in reclaiming your personal power after you have
experienced situations in which others tried to take your power
and control away from you.

MAGICAL USES

Not as aggressive in energy and nature as the warrior stone (garnet), the fire agate adds just enough "fire" to your determination that
you can break free of jealous, malicious, or greedy control by others.
Carry a piece of fire agate with you during the day and put it under
your pillow at night to sever any cordings caused by jealous co-
workers, ex-spouses, controlling parents, jealous so-called friends,
or nosey neighbors. The fire agate will break the cording with a
sharp, nasty little sting to the senders and keep them from reattach-
ing. Cording can draw off your energy as well as cause your home
environmental vibrations to turn sour, thus creating everything
from unusual excessive clumsiness to small accidents to streaks of
bad luck.

Fire agate is also useful when you need that extra little vitality and
poise when applying for a job, buying a car, facing and dealing with a
pushy attorney, or whenever you must confront a possible adversary.

Moss Agate

▶ **COLORS:** Moss agate is a translucent form of chalcedony, usually colorless, white, or gray. Within it are dark black, brown, red, or green moss or tree-like (dendritic) inclusions that give it its name.

▶ **SOURCES:** Moss agate is generally found in China, the U.S., and the Hindustan area of India. It is called moss agate, tree agate, and fern agate.

▶ **FACTS:** Another member of the chalcedony family, moss agate has branch-like or moss-like inclusions, which can be scattered randomly or appear in such a manner as to imitate a picture.

Moss agate is primarily cut in thin slabs or polished for mounting in jewelry.

▶ **HISTORY AND FOLKLORE:** Also known as Mocha Stone, moss agate got this name from an ancient source of the stone near the Arabian city of Mocha in Yemen. This stone is called *Piedra de Moca* in Spain, *Pierre de Mocka* in France, and *Mokkastein* in Germany. Because of its dendritic, or tree-like, inclusions, it is also known as tree agate.

The Greek Orpheus said that to wear moss agate was to receive divine favor and aid. Orpheus was so skilled a musician that it was said he could use his music to charm savage beasts or overcome death.

In Europe, farmers hung moss agate on fruit trees or from the horns of oxen when plowing so as to promote a bountiful crop. In the early 1800s, this stone was widely used in Europe and England as a luck ring. When it was worn as mourning jewelry symbolizing eternal life, it was surrounded with rubies.

Gypsies and people in the Orient prize moss agate because it is believed to make one eloquent and persuasive.

Moss agate is sometimes associated with Venus and Taurus, other times with Gemini.

To dream of moss agate signifies an increase in material comforts and prosperity.

▶ **HEALING ENERGIES:** Moss agate is one of the most powerful healing stones known. Place near the diseased portion of the body for rapid healing; especially good for wounds or after surgery. Has long been used to stop bleeding and begin the healing process. Balances and calms people who run on nervous energy. Said to relieve depression by balancing the two halves of the brain. This stone also cools and reduces both fever and temper. Wear to relieve a stiff neck.

▶ **MAGICAL POWERS:** Promotes moderation in life. Draws good health and long life; improves the vitality. Use as a touchstone to connect with Nature energies.

Moss agate is also a psychic stone, helping to develop, channel, and use the psychic abilities. Helps to create clarity of thought.

A stone that not only protects the aura, moss agate also aids in opening the third eye. Use for meditation, scrying, traveling the astral planes, and finding spirit guides. Useful when casting spells for wealth, happiness, long life, and to find new friends. Also said to help discover treasure.

MAGICAL USES

Beginners in the magical arts should carry or wear moss agate when practicing meditation, psychometry, telepathy, or any kind of divination. This not only gives added protection to the white light with which they surround themselves, but also makes it easier to access their budding psychic abilities.

Moss agate hung on a chain makes an excellent pendulum when map dowsing for a possible site for relocation or finding a new house or job. It is also often the most effective pendulum when learning how to dowse for water or underground lines of any kind.

Alabaster

▶ **HARDNESS:** 2

▶ **COLORS:** Usually white or gray; can be many other pastel shades.

▶ **SOURCES:** Italy and England.

▶ **FACTS:** A type of gypsum; a fine-grained, white translucent rock with a pearly luster. Primary use is in sculpturing.

▶ **HISTORY AND FOLKLORE:** Since alabaster has a tendency to erode quickly in damp climates, it was used mainly in the Middle East, Egypt, the Mediterranean, and the Far East. It was sculpted into statuary, vases, small jewelry boxes, perfume bottles, and ornate lamps. Alabaster was said to be favored by the Babylonian god Nin, son of Bel.

Unguent vases of alabaster have been found in ancient Egyptian tombs, including that of Tutankhamen. The tomb (dating c. 1500 B.C.E.) of a beautiful young woman held three such alabaster vases, among her other cosmetic containers.

Alabaster is associated with Venus and Taurus.

To dream of alabaster signifies a need to take more pride in yourself and your home.

▶ **HEALING ENERGIES:** None known.

▶ **MAGICAL POWERS:** Increases intellectual clarity. This stone can add confidence and an inner personal beauty that will improve your self-image.

MAGICAL USES

Keep a small piece of alabaster or an alabaster ornament or container with your daily beauty supplies, whether you are male or female. Its vibrations will permeate the supplies, plus the general area, so that you will take more pride in your personal appearance.

Alexandrite

▶ **HARDNESS:** 8.5

▶ **COLORS:** Natural alexandrite—purple-red that changes to green in daylight. Synthetic alexandrite—purple-red that changes to blue in daylight.

▶ **SOURCE:** Natural alexandrite of the best quality is found in the Ural Mountains in Russia.

▶ **FACTS:** This stone is a very rare and valuable variety of chrysoberyl, with the unusual phenomenon of changing color according to the light that strikes it. In daylight, this stone is an emerald green, but in artificial light, like a chameleon, it turns a raspberry red, mauve, or reddish brown.

Natural alexandrite can easily exceed $29,000 for a very small stone, if you could find one for sale. The alexandrite cat's-eye is even rarer and more costly. It is the most valuable of all chatoyant gemstones. There are very limited sources of this stone in Russia, Brazil, and Sri Lanka.

▶ **HISTORY AND FOLKLORE:** There is absolutely no mention of alexandrite in ancient writings. This stone was unknown until 1830, when it was discovered about sixty miles from Ekaterinburg, Russia on the birthday of Czar Alexander II; the stone was named in honor of the Czar. Its green and red colors were the same as the colors worn by the Imperial Guard.

Some writers list this as an Aquarian stone, while others put it under Scorpio.

To dream of alexandrite means struggle and progress.

▶ **HEALING ENERGIES:** Temporarily suspends tense emotional states.

▶ **MAGICAL POWERS:** Prevents other people from attaching cords to your astral body. Repels unwanted, undesirable people and energies. Helps with spiritual transformation and regeneration.

MAGICAL USES

Since this particular gem is far too expensive in its true form, consider purchasing a synthetic alexandrite instead. Wear or carry whenever you know you will be involved in any tense emotional situation; touch the stone often. If the situation occurs without your awareness, use the following spellworking as soon as possible afterward.

Set out dark blue and magenta candles, one each, in safe, metal candleholders. Either put these on your altar or in a place where they can burn completely out, undisturbed and safely. Carefully place one drop of patchouli oil on the wick end of the blue candle and one drop of lotus oil on the wick end of the magenta candle. Set them side by side with the alexandrite on the table between them. Burn lotus incense if you wish.

On a small piece of paper, briefly write out the details of the negative situation. Lay this paper under the holder containing the dark blue candle. On another small paper, write out the positive results you would like to see come from this situation, and lay it under the holder containing the magenta candle.

Light the dark blue candle and say: "I cannot erase what has happened, but I can change the outcome. By my will and desire a wall shall be built around the negative energy of this situation. As this candle burns away and dies, so shall the negative energy wither away to nothing."

Light the magenta candle and say: "This is my will and desire. With swiftness, the positive energy will grow and manifest. I am shielded from the negative and showered with the positive."

Touch the stone between the two candles and say: "This is my protector, the wall that allows only good to surround and affect me. This stone absorbs and changes for the better all negatives that touch it."

When the candles are burned out and completely cool, rip up the paper describing the negative situation. Throw it and the dark blue candle wax, if there is any left, into the garbage or bury it off your property. I prefer the garbage method, since this is an appropriate place for negatives. Set the alexandrite on the paper listing the positive outcomes you wish, and leave it there for seven days.

Amazonite

- ► **HARDNESS:** 6
- ► **COLOR:** Blue-green.
- ► **SOURCES:** India, the U.S., Canada, Russia, Madagascar, Tanzania, and Namibia. The best examples of this stone are said to be found near Pike's Peak in the U.S.
- ► **FACTS:** A semi-opaque microcline variety of feldspar, the color of amazonite can range from pale green to blue-green; it resembles some jades and opaque beryls. Its brilliant color is caused by the presence of lead. This semi-opaque stone is usually cut *en cabochon* for jewelry, but can be found in polished and unpolished pieces.
- ► **HISTORY AND FOLKLORE:** This stone does not come from the Amazon River area in South America. Amazonite was named after the Amazon River, according to one source, and after the Amazon women who worshipped the Moon goddess Diana, according to another.

It was known and used by the ancient Egyptians, Mesopotamians, and other ancient cultures of the Middle East. Pieces of jewelry now in museums have been dated back to the third millennium B.C.E.. In the ancient writings of Pliny there is a reference to the Assyrians associating this stone with their god Belus and using it in religious rituals. Pre-Columbian artifacts set with amazonite have also been found in Central and South America.

Amazonite is said to be under the signs of Virgo and Cancer.

To dream of amazonite symbolizes a struggle for independence.

▶ **HEALING ENERGIES:** Soothes the nervous system as it strengthens the heart and body.

▶ **MAGICAL POWERS:** Helps to align the mental and etheric bodies, thus giving clear vision of personal harmful tendencies and aiding in dispelling these. Can give creative inspiration, joy, and a desire to attain spiritually. Increases self-confidence; discourages destructive behavior.

Because this stone works well with the throat chakra, it can stimulate creativity and communication.

Good to use in rituals and celebrations of new life or new hope; also good for Beltane festivals.

MAGICAL USES

Men and women often embark on new cycles of life through changes in career, divorce, marriage, the birth of children, new goals, or important personality changes, to list just a few things. Amazonite set on your desk or near your bed will remind you, through its appearance and subtle vibrations, to hold tight to your decisions and celebrate the birth of the "new" in your life. This becomes especially important and helpful when the "new" has meant a painful and/or frightening decision.

When in need of calling forth your warrior spirit within, amazonite can help. By its very name, this stone evokes images of fiercely independent Amazon women warriors. Both men and women sometimes need the inner strength of their "warrior spirit" to not be bullied by controlling people or for the courage to step out into new areas of life.

A small piece of this stone, carried in the pocket or hung on a chain, can impart inner resolve and strength every time it is touched.

To realign the mental, emotional, astral, and spiritual bodies with the physical body, take a piece of amazonite in your power hand. Hold the stone over each of the chakras in turn, beginning with the root chakra just above the pubic bone and ending with the crown chakra at the top of the head. Do this slowly, while visualizing white light glowing around you.

Amber

▶ **HARDNESS:** 2.5

▶ **COLORS:** Yellow, orange, red, brown, gold; rarer and more expensive shades are violet, green, blue, and black.

▶ **SOURCES:** Baltic amber is gathered along the shores of the Baltic Sea, especially after great storms throw it up on the beaches. "Landlocked" amber, found in great swathes of "blue earth," is mined by the open-pit method using huge steam shovels.

Burmese amber ranges from red to brown in color and has a somewhat fluorescent appearance. It is found and mined only in an area near the jadeite mines in the Hukong Valley.

Sicilian amber is found around the mouth of the Simeto River in Sicily. It usually comes in the darker red hues. The Rumanian amber comes in even darker red shades, which can be almost black and shows fluorescence.

Amber is also found along the Samland Coast near Kalinigrad, Russia, as well as in Czechoslovakia, Germany, the Dominican Republic, Canada, and the U.S.

▶ **FACTS:** Amber is actually fossilized tree resin of extinct coniferous trees which lived about 120 million years old. Although usually a golden orange color, amber has been found in such rare shades as violet, green, blue, and black. It may be translucent or transparent, with a greasy shine. The cloudy appearance of amber comes from air spaces trapped inside when the resin solidified. On occasion, pieces of amber are discovered which contain insects, small arthropods, pieces of moss, lichens, and pine needles; these foreign inclusions were enveloped by the sticky resin before time and Nature transformed the resin into an organic "stone."

Amber is tough, but soft enough to carve or drill. True amber will float in a saturated salt solution, while amber substitutes will sink.

Most opaque, whitish or creamy amber seen in jewelry is really the golden-yellow that has been heated to give it that color. Cloudy amber is also heated in oil to fill the air spaces and make it transparent.

Amber was one of the first stones, or substances, to be used by very early humans in Asia, Africa, and Europe for amulets and decoration. Amber containing insects, leaves, and other foreign bodies has always had the highest value. One of the earliest mentions of amber in literature is in Homer's *Odyssey,* where it says that Eurymachus was given a necklace of amber beads. Trade in Baltic amber was a thriving business from the earliest of trading ventures. The Greeks knew the Baltic as the Amber Sea. An ancient Arabic tale tells of Amberabad ("Amber City") in Jinnistan ("fairy land").

Latin writers of the first century C.E. also mention its popularity. It was one of the most precious trading commodities between the cultures on the Baltic coast and those in the Mediterranean. When Schliemann excavated the graves in Mycenae, he discovered a considerable amount of Baltic amber. Amber carved in animal forms has also been found in tumuli in Indersoen, Norway.

Amber is one of the few stones that can be charged with electricity. When amber is rubbed briskly with cloth, it will attract small pieces of paper or hair. This property was known to the Greeks as early as the sixth century B.C.E. and accounts for the Greek name for amber—*elektron*—from which comes our modern word for electricity.

The gem world divides amber into four groups: Succinite (Baltic amber); Burmite (Burmese amber); Simetite (Sicilian amber); and Rumanite (Rumanian amber). The last three are the rarer forms and sources of this substance.

▶ **HISTORY AND FOLKLORE:** The name amber is probably derived from the Arabic word *ambar*. This stone was known to the Greeks as *succinum* ("juice or tree sap") and *elektron* ("electricity"), to the Oriental cultures as *karabe* ("straw attractor"), to the Romans as *amuletum*, and to the Hebrews as *hashmal*. The golden amber was called *chryselektrum* by the ancient writer Callistratus.

There are many beautiful and wondrous legends of the origin of amber around the world. The Norse said that it was formed from the goddess Freyja's tears falling into the sea. The ancient Greeks said that grains of amber were the petrified tears of the Heliades when they cried at the death of their brother Phaethon. Sophocles believed amber originated from the tears of certain Indian birds at the death of Meleager. In the writings of Pliny in the first century C.E. Rome, it was believed to be the solidified urine of the lynx, the darker from the male, the lighter from the female.[2] Two of the ancient writers, however, clarified this belief by stating that in Etruria a lynx was a tree and not an animal.[3] Another early writer called it the "juice" of the rays of the setting sun.

The Greek word for the gods' elixir of immortality was *ambrotos* (ambrosia), which was also linked with amber. This elixir was kept by the Goddess Hera, who also possessed the magical apples.[4] These apples are very similar to the story of the Norse goddess Siff and her golden apples of immortality.

Considered a protective stone, small pieces of amber were hung on the nets in the amphitheater to protect the podium from the wild animals. Gladiators used amber on their weapons and armor. Pliny wrote that carved amber was worth more than a healthy slave.[5]

For centuries, amber has been used in a variety of ways as medicine. Arab physicians used amber powder in many of their medicines. Pliny wrote that amber was good for tonsillitis and other throat infections. Powdered amber was given in wine for hysteria, as well as fever, croup, asthma, and hay fever. Finely powdered amber mixed with honey and rose oil was put into ears for earaches or ear infections. Roman physicians prescribed a mixture of amber powder and Attic honey, taken internally, for poor eyesight.

A similar mixture was also used for urinary problems, childbirth, loose teeth, and suppressed menses in women.

The use of amber for medicinal purposes was still being used by physicians well into the 1700s, when it was given for vertigo, asthma, arthritis, dysentery, fits, jaundice, scrofula, nervous afflictions, head colds, heart disease, and as a preventative of the plague.

Another early belief was that amber protected against evil sorcery and could counteract poisons. This repelling of poison still holds in many Eastern countries, where the mouthpieces of pipes and cigar and cigarette holders are made from amber so no infections are transmitted.

Oriental cultures used strings of amber beads to deepen and intensify meditation, thus helping one to reach a stronger enlightenment and become open to clairvoyance. The Chinese have an old tradition that says amber is made of the souls of dead tigers.

Apothecaries and medicine shops in many countries still carry prepared salts of amber to be made up into potions, lotions, and electuaries. A pungent oil distilled from amber is still known and used under the name of Oil of Succinate, or Oil of Amber. This mixture is rather like turpentine and is used extensively in preparing liniments.

Amber "Lammer beads" were considered a very effective charm to repel all kinds of evil, to protect against enchantment and bad luck, and to cure all types of diseases. These beads are still worn around the neck by many people in Scotland and Europe today. The late Shah of Persia wore a large piece of amber about his neck to protect against assassination.

Amulets carved in the forms of hares, dogs, fish, frogs, and lions were worn in Eastern Asia to make men virile and women fertile.

Although amber is often assigned to Cancer, Taurus, and Leo, it is also listed by some writers as belonging to Aquarius.

To dream of amber means a journey, movement, or change.

▶ **HEALING ENERGIES:** Wear around the neck to clear up chest problems, sore throats, bronchitis, asthma, and coughs. This stone has also been used to treat rheumatism, deafness, jaundice, headaches, goiter, bleeding teeth, and digestive problems. It's said to be especially beneficial when dealing with hysteria. It has high vibrations that can cleanse and purify the entire system and any of the bodies. Lighter colored amber is most useful for mental cleansing and healing, while the dark red helps most with regeneration healing. One tradition says to insert amber into the nostril to stop nosebleeds.

▶ **MAGICAL POWERS:** Healing, soothing, harmonizing. Helps to stabilize the kundalini and turns the intellect into more spiritual paths. Use it to increase the strength of spells and to attract money. Use on the altar to increase the strength of your magical spells.

Ambroid (amber pressed into forms; dark red-gold): calms fears and helps one keep an intellectual outlook.

Clear, dark red: will contain or destroy negative emotions; calms.

Clear golden brown: sharp intellectual focus; clears mental confusion; balances the sixth chakra.

Milky golden: same as clear, but with more inspirational energy.

Sea amber (another name is burnite; solid, dark golden brown): helps one stay neutral and realistic in difficult situations; balances the fifth chakra.

MAGICAL USES

Amber is such an attractive and beneficial organic stone that you will probably end up with more than one piece of it. Soothing to both the nerves and spirit, as well as imparting a sense of protection, amber jewelry is appropriate for wear at any time. Keep a piece on your altar or magical working space to bring in prosperity and add strength to every magical spellworking you do.

Ambroid, or pressed amber, is simply natural amber that has been carefully heated until soft, then pressed into molds. Often this amber appears in pyramid shapes; set this pyramid on top of a paper on which you have listed your desires for the week, month, or whatever time period you choose.

Amber pressed into a spherical shape has several magical and spiritual uses. Hold it while meditating on past lives. Its vibration can create a connection with your subconscious mind and thus open a pathway back to the appropriate lives that have a bearing, negatively or positively, on your present life. It can also be used during meditations to form a stronger link with your spiritual guides, thus enabling them to communicate what is needed for greater spiritual growth and expansion.

If you have a dark amber sphere, it can be used to heal sore muscles by rolling the ball slowly and gently over the sore area. You may experience mental visions of past times when doing this, times which may or may not have a connection with you.

Amethyst

▶ **HARDNESS:** 7

▶ **COLORS:** Shades and intensities of purple, lilac, and mauve. It can have a bluish or reddish purple tinge when viewed from different angles. Russian amethysts have a reddish tinge, while those from Canada are violet and those from Brazil a dark purple.

▶ **SOURCES:** Amethyst is found in the Ural Mountains in Russia, Canada, Sri Lanka, India, Uruguay, Brazil, Madagascar, the U.S., Germany, Australia, Nambia, Zambia, South Africa, and many other countries.

▶ **FACTS:** Amethyst is the most valuable form of quartz crystal. A few centuries ago, the most prized color was the deep-colored purple.

In the English Channel is the island of Sark. The people of this island are very fond of the amethyst, which is found there, and sell all of this stone under the name of "Sark stone."

The actor Patrick Swayze has an ancient foot-long braided silver wand, encrusted with gems and tipped with an amethyst. This wand is believed to be centuries old. Mr. Swayze uses this wand on discreet occasions for healing the sick and injured.

Crystals that are part citrine and part amethyst are known as ametrine. This is an authentic, Nature-made stone found only in Bolivia, South America. Ametrine is associated with the sign of Libra.

Some unscrupulous gem dealers heat amethyst, causing it to turn yellow, and then sell the altered stone as citrine.

► HISTORY AND FOLKLORE: Amethyst has long been prized as an ornament and amulet. Its most common ancient application was to prevent drunkenness. The word amethyst comes from the Greek word *amethystos*, meaning "non-intoxicating." Ancient Greeks and Roman wise men claimed that this stone, when dropped into a goblet of wine, neutralized the alcohol. This belief in the power of amethyst to prevent inebriation was still held in 1750, as reported by Camillus Leonardus, an Italian writer and physician to the Borgias. Leonardus also listed other powers of amethyst: represses evil thoughts; grants good understanding; makes a barren wife fruitful; gives victory to the military; and makes wild beasts and birds easy to capture.

This stone has a long history with religious practices. In the Egyptian *Book of the Dead*, instructions are given for placing heart-shaped amethysts on the body of the deceased. This use of the heart-shaped stone survives today in the practice of a groom giving one to his bride. Set in silver or gold, this uniquely cut stone is said to confer great happiness and tranquility to the newly married couple for the rest of their lives. It was also valued as a deterrent against burglars and intruders in the home.

It is quite possible that the Egyptians used the amethyst for other esoteric reasons, unknown to us today. We do know that scarabs were carved out of this stone and worn by soldiers as protective amulets against harm by weapons. The Chaldean Magi believed this stone protected against evil sorcery and brought success and good luck. Amethyst was also said to grant an understanding of hidden knowledge.

A story of the goddess Diana and the god Bacchus tells the Roman tale of the origin of amethyst. Bacchus, god of wine and good times, was furious because he felt neglected by mortals. He declared that his lions would devour the next human he met. Amethyst, a young maiden, crossed Bacchus' path on her way to Diana's shrine. When the lions began to tear at her, her screams caught the attention of Diana, who turned the girl into a pillar of transparent rock crystal. Bacchus became very contrite about his loss of control and, pouring wine over the pillar, turned its color from clear to purple.

At one time in China, pieces of amethyst were rented to people who were involved in lawsuits, for this stone was said to make one more positive in outlook, thus attracting a favorable outcome.

During the Middle Ages in Europe, amethyst was far more expensive than diamonds to purchase. Known then as the "bishop's stone," it was worn by cardinals and bishops. The Crusaders continued the Pagan use of amethyst by attaching it to their rosaries.

The wise men, magicians, and physicians of the Middle Ages believed that all bodily diseases were caused by a sickness of the soul. Combined with prayers to certain saints, they frequently recommended elixirs containing amethyst. Later, physicians used amethyst to cure headaches, toothaches, gout, insomnia, neuralgia, and protect against poisons and the plague. Francis Bacon (1561–1626 C.E.) wrote that, in his time, people still wore the amethyst and other precious stones for their ability to produce certain effects upon the body and the life.

Amethyst became extremely popular during the fifteenth century because it was thought to control and repel evil spirits. Soldiers wore it as an amulet against injury and death.

A very old custom recommended that an amethyst ring be worn on the third finger of the left hand in order to benefit fully from the stone's power; this practice was followed by medical practitioners for several centuries.

The amethyst has long been worn by sailors to ensure a safe journey and carried by soldiers as protection from harm.

Amethyst is said to be connected with Pisces, Virgo, Aquarius, and Capricorn and to be ruled by Jupiter. In Babylonian and Assyrian writings on astrology, the planet Jupiter, often associated with amethyst, was connected to the ninth house, or Sagittarius. Today, some writers assign amethyst to Jupiter while others associate it with Neptune.

To dream of amethyst symbolizes freedom from harm. It is also said that to dream of amethyst means your new undertakings will be very successful, especially if you are a traveler, sailor, philosopher, mystic, teacher, or of the clergy in one form or another.

▶ **HEALING ENERGIES:** The amethyst crystal is nearly indispensable for healers. Single crystals are very beneficial, but clusters are even more powerful and purifying. Because of this purifying power, amethyst clusters can be used to cleanse other stones; by placing the "soiled" stones on the cluster and leaving them there for at least 24 hours, the stones can be safely cleansed of any undesired or negative vibrations. If you use an amethyst cluster for this purpose, at least once a week soak it in a saline solution for 24 hours, rinse, and dry it carefully.

Amethyst calms mental disorders, purifies the blood, strengthens the immune system, and balances and heals all chakras. It is said to help physical pain, migraines, other headaches, insomnia, surgery, sore eyes, and psychological illnesses. For restlessness and insomnia, stroke the forehead and temples with a piece of amethyst. Its gentle energies will dispel tension and stress, as well as dissolve boredom.

To correct and balance the emotional and spiritual bodies, let the Moon shine through a piece of amethyst onto your crown chakra. To correct the physical body's energies and balance, let the Sun's rays shine through this stone onto the crown chakra. For healing a person who is not present, send your thoughts through the amethyst by holding it to your third eye.

▶ **MAGICAL POWERS:** Associated with the third eye, amethyst is often called the Spiritual Crystal. It is found in geodes, clusters, and single-pointed crystals. Its color can range from deep purplish blue to almost white. Sometimes this range of colors is found all in a single crystal. At least one writer relates amethyst to the third eye, or sixth chakra, while others assigned it to the crown, or seventh chakra.

Amethyst increases activity in the right brain (creative side), cuts through illusion, and helps to develop the psychic abilities. It is excellent for meditation as it strengthens and develops intuition, inspiration, healing, and channeling, as well as raising the thoughts and aspirations to a higher spiritual level. When worn on the left wrist, it enables one to foresee. Place with divination tools to strengthen their powers. Use in meditation to enhance psychic awareness.

Place under the pillow for pleasant dreams. If cut in a heart shape and given as a gift of love, amethyst will bring good fortune and happiness.

Amethyst promotes shrewdness in business matters, gives victory and preserves soldiers from harm, and quickens the mind and helps to control negative thoughts. Excellent for bringing good fortune in the fields of prophecy, writing, poetry, and publishing. Carry it to ensure justice in court cases.

Amethyst is very helpful in altering consciousness or switching levels, is said to encourage worship of the Goddess and God, and aids in creating a balance between the physical and spiritual.

Because this stone has transmutational energies, it helps to open gateways into intense and transforming spiritual experiences, and can protect the wearer from black magic. Known as a change stone, amethyst can bring about any type of change in your life and consciousness.

Ametrine (purple and yellow stripes): combining the old with new; excellent for those who have undergone an intense transformation.

Clear deep purple: connects with one's spiritual aspects; calms impatience and helps to pinpoint timing in a situation; promotes moderation in life; grounds during channeling.

Purple with white stripes: helps to balance soul friends.

Pale, opaque lavender (often sold as Cape Amethyst): relieves stress; aids in remembering, either past lives or early experiences in the present one; good for meditation, self-realization, and transformation.

MAGICAL USES

Wear amethyst set in a silver ring or silver bracelet on the left hand to open your psychic senses. This will sharpen your intuition, as well as helping you to develop your predictive abilities.

Exchanging gifts of heart-shaped amethysts between lovers will harmonize the vibrations between the two people, thus attracting a happy life and good fortune.

Wear or hold amethyst during meditation to help strength the communicative channels with your teachers or guides, or you can set an amethyst cluster or even part of an amethyst geode in the meditation area for the same effect.

Store a small piece of amethyst with your tarot cards or runes to keep the power of the divination tools high.

Although the use of no stone makes for instantaneous results, with patience, efforts are always rewarded.

Andalusite

▶ **HARDNESS:** 7.5

▶ **COLORS:** Varies from a pale yellowish brown to a dark bottle green, dark brown, or the most popular color, which is greenish red.

▶ **SOURCES:** Sri Lanka, Brazil, Spain, Canada, Russia, Australia, and the U.S.

▶ **FACTS:** Andalusite can be found in either opaque, rod-like crystals or waterworn pebbles. The pebbles are the pieces ordinarily cut as gemstones. This stone has strong pleochroism, which means that when turned, it can appear yellow, green, and red.

One variety, an opaque, yellowish gray occurs in long prisms. These are rare. They are cut in cross-sections to show the cross formation inside.

Another variety of andalusite is chiastolite. This name comes from the Greek word *chiastos* ("marked with an X," or the letter chi). This is a cross stone, whose design appears when cross sections of chiastolite are cut. These polished sections are worn or carried as amulets.

▶ **HISTORY AND FOLKLORE:** None known.

Andalusite is associated with the element of Earth.

To dream of this stone symbolizes an upcoming task that will require all your attention and energy if you are to get through it successfully.

▶ **HEALING ENERGIES:** Unknown.

▶ **MAGICAL POWERS:** Creates an aggressive, dynamic energy for accomplishing large and long-term projects; promotes success; keeps one completely focused on the task at hand.

MAGICAL USES

Place a piece of andalusite beside the candle when doing candle-burning spells. This will concentrate and strengthen the magical energy. Double its effect by using a magenta candle along with the appropriate spell candle.

Wrap this stone in a small piece of dark green cloth and carry in your left-hand pocket, or pin inside your lingerie on the left side. This helps bring in innovative ideas, strength, and will power when working on a long-term project that requires you to be on your toes at all times.

Apatite

► **HARDNESS:** 5

► **COLORS:** Colorless, yellow, blue, violet, or green.

► **SOURCES:** Myanmar, Sri Lanka, Brazil, Russia, Canada, East Africa, Sweden, Spain, and Mexico.

► **FACTS:** Apatite can be opaque to transparent and occurs in hexagonal prisms or tabular crystals. The blue from Myanmar is strongly dichroic, meaning it is colorless when viewed from one direction and blue when viewed from another, much like aquamarine. Blue apatite, both from Myanmar and Sri Lanka, can be cut *en cabochon* to show a cat's eye because of fibrous inclusions. Chatoyant stones are also found in Brazil; some of these are yellow or green. "Asparagus stone" is actually Spanish apatite of a yellowish green color. A blue-green variety, called moroxite, is found in Norway.

Named for the Greek word for deception, apatite imitates in its chemical composition many other stones.[6] In fact, about 65 percent of mammalian teeth and bones are made up of this stone.

► **HISTORY AND FOLKLORE:** None known.

Apatite is associated with the sign of Gemini by some writers.

To dream of apatite means something will occur psychically that will alert you to the beginning of a new cycle in your life.

▶ **HEALING ENERGIES:** Balances the emotions.

▶ **MAGICAL POWERS:** Continued use of apatite can produce a spiritual state of unconditional love. Apatite creates a willingness to let go of useless aspects of life, people, or objects. It enhances psychic abilities and creativity.

MAGICAL USES

Apatite is very useful when you are having difficulty letting go of someone or something that no longer is good for you or has a place in your life. Hold a piece of apatite and meditate for five minutes a day for seven days. Each day, during this meditation, visualize yourself pushing the person or problem farther away from you. By the end of a week, you will find you have better control over your emotions that once tied you to this inappropriate person or problem.

Aquamarine

▶ **HARDNESS:** 7.5–8

▶ **COLORS:** Shades of light blue, sky blue, bluish green, watery green.

▶ **SOURCE:** Brazil, the Urals and Siberia in Russia, Afghanistan, Pakistan, India, Nigeria, and Madagascar.

▶ **FACTS:** A member of the beryl family of stones, aquamarine is dichroic, which means that the stone appears blue when viewed from one direction and colorless when seen from another. Gem-quality aquamarine has been found up to 39 inches long and flawless. The best stones come from Brazil, where it is known as *cascalho*. A dark blue variety comes from Madagascar.

Gem dealers have never been able to successfully duplicate or synthesize aquamarine.

▶ **HISTORY AND FOLKLORE:** The name aquamarine comes from the Latin words *aqua* (water) and *mare* (the sea), and the gemstone does indeed remind one of the light color of seawater.

This stone is held in high regard in the East as the Stone of the Seer and Mystic, a gem that imparts purity to the wearer.

A large aquamarine once adorned the crown of James II of

England. However, when the crown-stones were later valued, it turned out to be only a piece of glass. No one is certain how or when the real stone was replaced.

Kozminsky[7] states that the aquamarine and the entire beryl family are associated with the sign of Taurus, because their crystalline form is hexagonal (six-sided) and six is a number belonging to Venus. Other writers say it is connected with Gemini, Pisces, and Aries.

To dream of an aquamarine means loving friendships, happy relationships, and pleasant social activity.

▶ **HEALING ENERGIES:** Aquamarine is said to help eliminate fluid retention by strengthening the kidneys, liver, spleen, and thyroid, thus purifying the body. It calms the nerves and also heals diseases in the eyes, throat, and stomach. At one time, eyeglasses were made of aquamarine because this stone is soothing to the eyes.

▶ **MAGICAL POWERS:** Clears the mind and aids creativity. Balances the emotions. Can aid in banishing fears, doubts, and phobias, while helping you to become more tolerant and take responsibility for your life and actions. Changes vacillation into inner authority.

Good for meditation as it brings calmness, peace, inspiration, and love. Strengthens personal power and the aura. Aids in taking control of any situation where one must be powerful.

This stone is very helpful when facing a court case or litigation; protects against unjust enemies. Can bring marriage partners back together after separations. Carried, it protects from accidents and attracts wealth.

Known as the mystic and seer's stone, aquamarine has a balancing effect on all the bodies; its vibrations are subtle and long lasting. Excellent for purification of the emotions, mind, and spirit. Sharpens the intuition, while quieting a restless mind. Also said to open communications with water entities.

MAGICAL USES

Although aquamarine has a wide range of uses, its strongest energies are in the field of opening up the psychic. Wearing this stone sensitizes the subconscious mind, sometimes breaking down mental barriers and allowing psychic impressions to flood through. If you are especially sensitive to the thoughts and vibrations of other people, wear aquamarine with smoky quartz. This combination will ease the sharpness of incoming psychic impressions, while the smoky quartz will also ground you in the physical. In this way, you can avoid being swamped by unwanted impressions.

Aventurine

- ▶ **HARDNESS:** 7
- ▶ **COLORS:** Usually green; the types of inclusions alter the shade. Can also be dark red through peach to brown.
- ▶ **SOURCES:** Brazil, India, Russia, the U.S., Australia, Germany, Japan, and Tanzania.
- ▶ **FACTS:** A type of quartz, aventurine has sometimes been confused with aventurine feldspar, amazonite, and jade. Aventurine is also sometimes called Indian jade, which is a misnomer, although the bright green stones are almost as valuable as jade. It should not be confused with aventurine feldspar, which is a red variety of albite. The true green aventurine has fuchsite mica inclusions, while the greenish brown has goethite and the brown has pyrite. It is presently understood that the name aventurine is applied to the green colored stone.

  The name was derived from a type of glass made in Italy, which was said to have been discovered by mistake (*a ventura*).
- ▶ **HISTORY AND FOLKLORE:** None known. This stone is often associated with Aries.

  To dream of aventurine means a change of circumstances or life cycle that brings with it less anxiety about the future.
- ▶ **HEALING ENERGIES:** Aventurine can relieve anxiety and fear. Has strong healing energy that affects the pituitary gland. Soothes the eyes and relieves migraines.
- ▶ **MAGICAL POWERS:** Use to release anxieties and build positive attitudes, good health, and independence. Excellent when working to

center yourself. Has a direct channel to Earth energy, thus making it easier to balance and calm. Balances male and female energies.

A protective stone, aventurine repels anxiety and fear while encouraging positive attitudes. Scott Cunningham, in *Cunningham's Encyclopedia of Crystal, Gem and Metal Magic,* recommends it as a good luck piece for gambling.

Since this stone can enhance creative visualization, it is excellent for writers, artists, musicians, or anyone in the creative fields.

Used with malachite, it can help to clear out mental or emotional blockages. Used with rose quartz, aventurine will increase empathic qualities.

Green: enhances self esteem; keeps sixth and seventh chakras open; creates harmony and balance; helps in channeling. Makes a powerful good luck piece that will draw opportunities your way. Can also draw unexpected adventures and good luck in love. Can aid in purifying the mental, emotional, and etheric bodies.

Red: stimulates creativity and communications; keeps second through fifth chakras open; balances all the bodies.

MAGICAL USES

Although green aventurine will attract prosperity and love, it also draws unexpected adventures or incidents. If you are the timid or shy type of person, you might find this unsettling. However, if you persevere, this stone can help you overcome shyness.

To attract prosperity specifically, write out your desires on a small piece of paper. Put one drop of honeysuckle oil on the center of the paper, fold it four times, and then place it in a little cloth bag with the aventurine. Carry this in your pocket or purse.

Azurite

▶ **HARDNESS:** 3.5–4
▶ **COLORS:** Azure to navy blue, sometimes with bands of green malachite.
▶ **SOURCES:** Australia, Chile, Russia, Africa, France, and China.

▶ **FACTS:** A massive blue opaque, copper mineral that has intergrown with malachite. The stones found near Chessy, France are called chessylite.

Azurite is frequently found mixed with other minerals. For example, azurmalachite or burnite is a combination of azurite and cuprite (copper oxide). One of the few truly blue minerals, polished pieces of azurite mixtures have beautiful patterns.

▶ **HISTORY AND FOLKLORE:** Azurite has been in use by ancient Middle Eastern cultures for nearly as long as lapis lazuli. Ancient Egyptian priestesses and priests used azurite to raise the consciousness to such a high level that they could contact the Goddess.

This stone is connected with the sign of Sagittarius by some writers.

To dream of azurite symbolizes a truth soon to be revealed.

▶ **HEALING ENERGIES:** Strengthens the blood and the flow of energy through the nervous system. This stone has a light cleansing and purifying effect on the body and mind.

▶ **MAGICAL POWERS:** Enhances the psychic, but cuts through illusion to the truth. Aids in having clear meditations and working toward self-transformations. If you do not want to experience a transformation, avoid using azurite, for it will act as a catalyst.

Enhances creativity, inspiration, intuition. Aids in confidence and spiritual cleansing. Useful when studying for exams as it helps to retain information.

A symbol of the eye of spirit, azurite helps to unlock other dimensions of being. Use on the third eye during meditation for spiritual awareness and higher wisdom. Aids in removing blockages to psychic powers, especially clairvoyance, by energizing the third eye and expanding the inner vision.

MAGICAL USES

Place a piece of azurite on your desk or working space when studying for a class, doing research, or brainstorming for project ideas.

If you desire to do deep meditations or astral travel across time and space, tape this stone to the center of your forehead over the third eye.

I do not recommend doing this more often than once in ten days time, as the too frequent use of azurite this way tends to make you spacey.

Barite

▶ **HARDNESS:** 3

▶ **COLORS:** A variety of colors, including colorless, white, yellow, and blue.

▶ **SOURCES:** Cornwall and Derbyshire in England, Czechoslovakia, Romania, Germany, the U.S., and Italy.

▶ **FACTS:** A very brittle stone, barite is never cut for jewelry. Its name means "heavy." Because it is tasteless, odorless, harmless to the digestive system, and opaque to X rays, powdered barite is the main ingredient in barium solutions used to get pictures of the stomach or intestines.

The crystals can be opaque to transparent, as well as anything from massive formation to tabular crystals. It is commonly found in lead and silver mines, and can be seen deposited by hot springs. The largest crystals (up to 40 inches) have been discovered in Cornwall and Derbyshire, England.

One form of barite tabular crystal is called Desert Rose or Celunite Rose. This naturally formed mineral resembles a rose with all its petals. The flat barite plates were filled with sand during formation, resulting in this unusual and beautiful rosette.

Never cleanse with water!

▶ **HISTORY AND FOLKLORE:** None known.

The Desert Rose is associated with the element of Earth.

To dream of ordinary barite signifies an imbalance in the body and possible upcoming illness. To dream of Desert Rose, however, means a new friendship that could crumble into nothing if not handled gently.

▶ **HEALING ENERGIES:** Said to be good for concentrating more calcium into the bones, especially in women.

▶ **MAGICAL POWERS:** Useful in establishing contact with Nature spirits.

MAGICAL USES

If you want to contact the Nature spirits who are responsible for your garden or house plants, place a Desert Rose, a piece of ginger root, and a brown candle on a small tray. Powdered ginger can be substituted for the root.

Light the candle and say: "I wish to speak with all those beings who protect and help my garden and plants. I bid you welcome within my home and thank you for all your efforts."

Sit quietly before the burning candle for several minutes. The Nature spirits often make their presence known by small, swift movements seen from the corners of your eyes. If you have cats or dogs, these animals may acknowledge the spirits' presence by watching their movements or playing with them.

Extinguish the candle at the end of your vigil, and save it for another time. Once you have established communication with these Nature guardians, do not be surprised if they move into your home during the winter months when your outside plants are dormant.

Beryl

▶ **HARDNESS:** 7.5

▶ **COLORS:** Red, green, yellow.

▶ **SOURCES:** The red is found in the Thomas Mountains and Wah Wah Mountains in Utah. Yellow and green are found in or near emerald mines.

▶ **FACTS:** A very rare stone and seldom cut, red beryl is also called bixbite. It has an intense red color due to manganese. It has a hexagonal crystal structure and is usually attached to a matrix of other stone. The green (not emerald) and yellow beryls are often found in the vicinity of emerald mines, but are usually cast aside as having little importance.

On very rare occasions, beryl cat's-eye and star stones are found. A raspberry red beryl is mined in Utah under the name of bixbite; however, most specimens are badly flawed.

▶ **HISTORY AND FOLKLORE:** The name beryl comes from either the

Greek and Latin word *beryllus* or the Persian *belur*. Even in Pliny's time, people were aware that certain valuable stones, such as emerald, belonged to the beryl family.

Greek physicians treated bladder and kidney stones by dipping a beryl in water and then giving the water to the patient to drink. This stone was widely known for healing and divination in ancient societies.[8]

During the Middle Ages, beryl was used in a specific divination ritual, using the stone and a bowl of water. The beryl was suspended on a chain or string and held over the bowl, just barely touching the surface of the water. When a question was asked, the stone would strike the sides of the bowl. Beryl was also placed in a shallow dish of water; when sunlight shone in the water, the reflections would produce visions.

Also during this period of history, beryl was called the *Panzoon* ("All Life") in a book published in 1685.[9] If engraved with the image of a hoopoe bird, this stone was thought to invoke the spirits of the dead.[10]

An old tradition says that wearing beryl will make a lazy person more industrious and one slow of wits smarter.

This stone is associated with Neptune and Pisces.

To dream of beryl means good news is coming.

▶ **Healing Energies:**
Gold: helps with allergies to plants and pollens.
Green: beryl is useful in treating eye and throat diseases.
White: helps with dust allergies.
Yellow: can be applied for liver problems and jaundice.

▶ **Magical Powers:** A symbol of undying youth, beryl can be used ritually to strengthen the memory and produce new, innovative thoughts. Said to cure laziness, as well as finding hidden things.

Will increase psychic awareness and divination abilities. For scrying, no stone is supposed to be as powerful and effective as beryl. In fifth century Ireland scryers used beryl spheres for this purpose.

Use in rituals to bring rain.

Beryl also has a long tradition of preventing psychic manipulation. If you think about this carefully, you will recognize such actions are common in everyday life, particularly by salespeople, ranting fanatics in all areas, including religion, the news media, and of course, politics.

Colorless: breaks down stubbornness and rigidity.

Pale green: aids listening as well as communicating; stabilizes energy levels.

Pale yellow to green-yellow: helps one to avoid being tagged or corded (see below).

Pink, pale violet, strawberry red: helps to break down prejudices and intolerance.

MAGICAL USES

The vibrational energy from this stone is low key and slow acting. It is excellent, however, for people who feel uncomfortable with the more energetic stones.

If you are being tagged or corded by certain people, tape a small piece of tumbled beryl over your navel. Tagging or cording is when another person attaches an astral line to your astral body (usually in the area of the third chakra); through this cord they can drain your energy and even manipulate your actions, if they are determined enough.

Bloodstone

▶ **HARDNESS:** 7

▶ **COLORS:** Green with red flecks.

▶ **SOURCES:** India, Brazil, China, Australia, and the U.S.

▶ **FACTS:** A form of chalcedony, which is actually an opaque green jasper with red flecks or spots. Its old name (Heliotrope) comes from two Greek words—*helios*, the Sun, and *tropos*, to turn. It came from the belief that a bloodstone immersed in water would capture the sun as a blood-red image. Pliny mentioned that the same procedure was used to capture the image of a solar eclipse.

▶ **HISTORY AND FOLKLORE:** Rings of bloodstone were popular among the ancient Egyptians. They liked to wear such rings on the thumb, perhaps because the thumb is said to be under the influence of

Mars, which is the ruling planet of Aries. One such Egyptian ring was in the form of a dragon surrounded by sunrays. The *Leyden Papyrus* says that this stone will open any door and break down walls.

The Greeks and Romans wore bloodstone for a number of reasons: to gain endurance during athletics, to secure the favor of those in power, to bring renown, and to protect against the bites of poisonous scorpions, snakes, and other creatures. The later Gnostics believed that this stone prolonged life and brought wealth.

Ancient physicians called the bloodstone *Lapis Sanguinarius*. They said it stopped the flow of blood from wounds and hemorrhages as well as helping with hemorrhoids. Chinese doctors used bloodstone set in gold to stop nosebleeds and prevent the formation of kidney stones.

Leonardus, physician to the Borgias, wrote that if this stone was rubbed with the juice of the plant heliotrope it would make the wearer invisible; he also said that bloodstone rendered poisons harmless and gave safety and long life to the owner. Francis Barrett (1801) wrote much the same, adding that this stone could make the wearer famous. It was also believed to cause thunder, lightning, and storms.

From the Middle Ages, various sculptors carved the head of their Christ in bloodstone so the red flecks matched the places on the head torn by the crown of thorns. This practice was connected with a legend that said Christ's blood at the crucifixion splashed onto dark green jasper, thus producing the bloodstone.

Traditionally, bloodstone is said to predict the future by causing meteorological extremes, such as winds, storms, thunder, and lightning, to appear to announce the coming event.

It is said you can enhance its powers by placing it in water and setting the water in direct sunlight.

This stone is often connected with Aries and Mars.

Bloodstone in a dream means the arrival of distressing news.

▶ **HEALING ENERGIES:** Helps with physical and mental energy by cleansing the blood and any organs connected with the blood; can detoxify the body. A powerful physical healer, it reduces mental and emotional stress. An excellent healing stone that initiates renewal on all levels, bloodstone helps in overcoming depression and emotionally caused pain. The *Leyden Papyrus* says that this stone can be used in treatment of tumors and growths.

▶ **MAGICAL POWERS:** Since this stone tends to link the root and heart chakras, thus stimulating the kundalini, use it with caution.

Guards the owner against deceptions and being cheated and preserves the health. Creates a high prosperity consciousness and a willingness to accept abundance. Strengthens self-confidence and opens the senses to inner guidance.

Also said to lengthen life, give fame, bring money, and aid you in being unnoticed when you desire. The ancient Egyptians used bloodstone as a charm to acquire any desired thing, tear down all walls to success, dispel the wrath of authorities, and make all words believable.

Helps the magician gain control over negative spirits and to cast spells. Aids in foretelling the future and causing storms.

MAGICAL USES

As with any type of magic, you have no right to try to deliberately control another person, nor is the eventual backlash from such action worth the effort. However, if you are in the right (not just your opinion you are) or are sincerely desiring to take responsibility for wrong actions and make a new start in life, bloodstone can help. If faced with a court case or lawsuit, lay the bloodstone on the official papers and leave it there for three nights. Meditate for five minutes each night on the positive changes and actions you plan to take. Be sincere, because if you are merely attempting to get off the hook and do not regret what you did wrong, the energy of this stone will backfire on you in the near future. Carry the bloodstone with you when you go into court.

Boji Stones

▶ **HARDNESS:** 7.4
▶ **COLORS:** A nondescript brown or tan.

▶ **SOURCE:** The U.S.

▶ **FACTS:** A fairly new stone to magicians, metaphysicians, and rock collectors, the Boji stones are still in the process of being studied for their healing and magical effects. The couple who have marketed the Boji stones since 1972[11] have created an aura of mystery around these strange rocks. According to their literature, the Boji stones are said to come from around the bottom of a natural pyramid-shaped mountain, somewhere in an arid section of the middle of the United States. This area is thought to have been held sacred by Native Americans.

Said to grow on stems that are uncovered by erosion, Bojis appear to be a strange type of fossil-rock. They are small and rather round or ovoid in shape. If the Boji's energy is destroyed or depleted, it changes from hard rock to dust, a type of decaying more like plants or animals. Sold in pairs, the smooth stone is called female and the rough stone with angular projections, male.

▶ **HISTORY AND FOLKLORE:** None available.

Boji stones are associated with the element of Earth.

To dream of these stones reveals a need to balance your male and female energies.

▶ **HEALING ENERGIES:** Relieves or lessens pain and speeds healing. If kept near you part of the time each day, the Bojis will aid in releasing fear, a prime cause of some illnesses. Use the male stone on the left side of the body, the female stone on the right side.

▶ **MAGICAL POWERS:** Use these stones to close any holes in the human aura and to cut any attached cordings from others. This process has been shown through Kirlian photography.

MAGICAL USES

When using the Boji stones, hold one in each hand and move them toward each other until you feel a slight magnetic attraction or repulsion. If you do not feel this, turn one of the stones and try again. It may take a few tries until you experience the very slight magnetic movement. These stones are not magnetic, as are lodestones; the energy force you feel is psychic polarity.

When using to break cordings or close holes in the aura, take the male stone in your left hand and the female in your right. Run your hands a few inches away from the physical body, both hands moving at the same time. Use slow, gentle sweeping movements. After completely sweeping the entire aura, give the stones a rest for several hours before repeating the procedure.

Bronzite

- ► **HARDNESS:** 5.5
- ► **COLORS:** Greenish brown with a bronze-like luster.
- ► **SOURCE:** Austria.
- ► **FACTS:** Bronzite is part of the same series of minerals as enstatite. It is the iron-bearing variety and has many inclusions that give it a greenish brown, bronze-like luster. Slightly dark and brittle, bronzite is seldom used in jewelry, although it is cut *en cabochon* for collectors.
- ► **HISTORY AND FOLKLORE:** None known.

    Bronzite is associated with Venus and Taurus.

    To dream of bronzite symbolizes important changes that are coming your way.
- ► **HEALING ENERGIES:** Helps with loosening up stiff muscles.
- ► **MAGICAL POWERS:** Opens and balances third chakra; stimulates the desire to exercise and move in life.

    Helpful when planning physical moves, such as to another home or occupation, especially if a great distance is involved.

MAGICAL USES

If you have a house or property in mind to rent or purchase, and are unsure if someone else might beat you to it, take a picture of the house or land. Put this picture in a place where it will not be disturbed for at least seven days. Set a piece of bronzite on top of this picture. Every day, for at least fifteen minutes, sit quietly and visualize yourself living there. This will increase your opportunities for getting your desire.

Calcite

▶ **HARDNESS:** 3

▶ **COLORS:** Colorless, pink, green, orange, black, blue, brown, gray, red, violet.

▶ **SOURCES:** Common worldwide. Italy, Germany, England, the U.S., and Iceland for Iceland Spar.

▶ **FACTS:** The principal component of limestone and marbles, calcite is also found in large, transparent crystals intergrown with other minerals. It is also found in many stalactites and stalagmites. The famous creamy Carrara marble of Italy is composed of calcite.

The transparent, colorless Iceland Spar, with its white fibrous form, is cut *en cabochon,* to show chatoyancy, or cat's-eye qualities. Iceland Spar was first found in Iceland and was originally used to make polarizing prisms. Anything viewed through Iceland Spar is seen as a double image.

▶ **HISTORY AND FOLKLORE:** None known.

Clear calcite is connected with the Moon and Cancer; pink, blue, and green with Venus and Taurus; orange with the Sun and Leo.

To dream of pink or blue calcite symbolizes a birth or new beginnings. Orange calcite in dreams means to be alert for events or people who may push you into something you will later regret. Green calcite signifies opportunities to better oneself.

▶ **HEALING ENERGIES:**

Green: helps to clear toxic damage from the body and environment.

▶ **MAGICAL POWERS:**

Black: aids one in clearly seeing the truth, no matter what it is; helps in making plans to cover all aspects of a situation.

Blue: balances the emotional state; removes blockages; balances and heals all chakras. Cunningham recommends placing blue calcite between two purple or blue candles for healing spells.

Brown or gold: intensifies clarity of life and events.

Gray: temporarily neutralizes karmic influences.

Green: attracts money and prosperity into the home.

Orange: reduces skepticism; protects.

Pink: grounding; use in love rituals.

Red: helps to drain negative emotions from the body and mind; balances the fourth chakra.

Violet: creates peace and harmony.

White or clear: helps with spiritual awareness; balances the seventh chakra; aids in self-love and feeling worthy; good for meditation.

MAGICAL USES

Calcite is excellent for use in candle-burning rituals. Choose the color of the calcite and candles to match your desired result. Lay the calcite between two candles, then leave it there while the candles burn out.

Carnelian

▶ **HARDNESS:** 7

▶ **COLORS:** Orange, reddish orange, brownish red.

▶ **SOURCES:** Most carnelian today comes from Campo de Maia in South America. It is also found in Warwick, England, Queensland, Australia, and Ratnapura, India, which has the finest carnelian.

▶ **FACTS:** A form of brownish red or reddish orange chalcedony. Part of the same group as sard, bloodstone, moss agate, banded agate, and chrysoprase. Carnelian is very sensitive, especially to oils and acids.

▶ **HISTORY AND FOLKLORE:** This stone has been known for many centuries, and its name is said to come either from the Kornel cherry or the Latin word *carnis* (flesh, as in its color). In old Roman writings, the darker colors were said to be male, the lighter shades female. The ancient people knew that exposing carnelian to the Sun's rays would brighten their color; this intensification of color cannot be obtained through the use of ordinary heat.

Ancient cultures used carnelian in medicine, magic, and practical affairs. Because carnelian will separate easily from wax or clay, it was widely used by merchants, kings, and the upper classes in seal rings. During the Middle Ages, men wore carnelian to prevent enchantment. Throughout the Middle East carnelian was, and still is, worn as protection against the evil eye, which is said to be able to make one lose one's fortune.

The ancient Egyptians called carnelian the "blood of Isis" and wore it for protection as well as placing it on the throat of the deceased at the time of embalming. It was especially popular among the followers of Isis, who believed it acted as a talisman for protection when traveling through the Underworld after death. They carved the carnelian into many magical shapes, the most popular being the buckle of Isis and the heart amulet called the *ab*. One chapter of the *Book of the Dead* is devoted to the carnelian buckle of this goddess.

In Arabia and Turkey, the dark red carnelians are the ones most prized and thought to be the most powerful. Moslems call this the Mecca stone and believe it fulfills all desires, thus bringing perfect happiness. Mohammed is said to have worn a carnelian ring as an amulet for a blessed life after death.[12]

In some Oriental cultures this stone is believed to protect from evil sorcery, prevent ill health and the plague, and ward off the envious.

The ancients believed that carnelian was good for combating bad temper. Since bad temper was thought to be caused by black magic, the onset of such could be determined by watching for an unusual sheen over the surface of any carnelian worn for protection. It was also considered valuable as a deterrent to hemorrhage, nosebleeds, hard menstruation, and bleeding wounds.

Ancient physicians had other healing uses for carnelian besides stopping bleeding. They prescribed it powdered in a drink against fluxes and bound it to the belly of birthing women to aid the progress of childbirth. It was also recommended for treating jaundice. Carried or worn, carnelian was said to give courage and dispel fear, defend the body against all poisons, create a cheerful mind, and prevent unwanted fascinations.

If placed in front of a light and gazed at intently, this stone was said to help in astral travel. H. P. Blavatsky wrote in her book, *Isis Unveiled*, of Tartar shamans who carried a carnelian under their left arm to aid in astral travel and also to do strong magic.

The rare yellow carnelian is linked to the Sun, while the orangish tints are connected with the sign of Leo.

If you dream about carnelian, evil thoughts are being directed against you; beware of possible misfortune.

▶ **HEALING ENERGIES:** This stone has strong, beneficial electromagnetic properties. Strengthens and energizes the blood and all organs connected with the blood. Also helps to regenerate damaged tissue. Strengthens a weak voice.

Carnelian has long been used to stop blood flow; it is placed on the back of the neck for a nosebleed. It is also useful in easing menstrual cramps and is excellent for lower back trouble. This stone is also a traditional healing treatment for shrinking tumors.

▶ **MAGICAL POWERS:** Use in rituals to speed manifestation. Revitalizes and aligns the physical, mental, emotional, and spiritual bodies.

Aids in understanding the inner self and strengthens concentration. Helps overcome the fear of speaking in public. Increases the sense of self-worth. Carnelian is excellent for career success; fast acting. Keep nearby when studying, as carnelian stimulates the concentration and memory. Balances creative and organizational abilities. Opens doors and creates a need to follow through on plans.

Protects from ill-wishing; drives away evil. Protects against collapsing buildings; brings good luck. Wear this stone to prevent other people from reading your thoughts or dark forces from influencing the mind.

Helps to heal family problems. Use to remember astral travels or connect with past historical events.

MAGICAL USES

Wear carnelian around the neck to overcome shyness and to help when speaking in public. Wear in a ring on the left hand to remember astral travels or when checking into past lives. Wear on the right hand as protection from cording. Place near a window as an alarm for approaching storms or disasters.

Cassiterite

- ▶ **HARDNESS:** 6.5
- ▶ **COLORS:** Usually brilliant black; also yellow, pale brown, reddish brown.
- ▶ **SOURCES:** Malay Peninsula, England, Germany, Australia, Bolivia, Mexico, and Namibia.
- ▶ **FACTS:** The principal ore of tin, cassiterite crystals are usually short and stubby. They can easily be confused with diamond, brown zircon, and titanite. However, they have a distinct dichroism, different colors when viewed from different angles, and frequently have black mineral inclusions. The name cassiterite comes from the Greek word *kassiteros*, which means tin.

    Although cassiterite is a metal ore, it does not look metallic. The crystals are shiny and translucent, instead of dull and opaque.
- ▶ **HISTORY AND FOLKLORE:** None known.

    Cassiterite is associated with Mercury and Gemini.

    To dream of this stone means you need to stop procrastinating and get things in your life in order.
- ▶ **HEALING ENERGIES:** Unknown.
- ▶ **MAGICAL POWERS:** Helps with organizational and strategic skills; makes one more productive, focused, and forceful.

MAGICAL USES

Everyone should have a list of proposed future goals for her/his life. If you are growing and expanding as you should, this list will be revised from time to time. Placing cassitterite on top of this list will attract ideas and opportunities that are appropriate for you.

Cat's-Eye

- ▶ **HARDNESS:** 8.5 (cymophane, or chrysoberyl cat's-eye)
- ▶ **COLOR:** Fairly transparent and usually greenish yellow, gray-green, yellow, or grayish yellow with chatoyancy properties when cut *en*

cabochon. The most expensive color of chrysoberyl cat's-eye is a light golden or honey brown, often with a shadow that produces a light and dark effect. The chatoyancy is caused by numerous fine, parallel crystal needles.

▶ **Sources:** Found in Sri Lanka, Brazil, Ceylon, and China.

▶ **Facts:** A type of chrysoberyl with feather-like fluid inclusions or needle-like inclusions of rutile, this version of the cat's-eye has the longest history of all the chrysoberyls. It was already well known in Rome at the end of the first century. After the Duke of Connaught gave a cat's-eye betrothal ring to his fiancée in the late nineteenth century, the popularity and price of this stone rose considerably. The name chrysoberyl comes from the Greek words *chrysos* ("golden") and *beryllos* (which refers to the beryllium content of the stone).

The finest specimens of cymophane come from Ceylon, where they have long been used as a charm against evil spirits. Ceylon cat's-eyes are also rare and extremely expensive; a small cabochon the diameter of the tip of the little finger can easily bring $5,000 to $7,000. Sources of this stone are now scarce, because it has been nearly mined out, as has its relative the alexandrite. It is harder than a topaz and, correctly cut, has an opalescent gleam.

For quartz cat's-eye, see Crocidolite.

▶ **History and Folklore:** Known for thousands of years in the Orient, chrysoberyl cat's-eye stones were highly valued as the best repellant of the evil eye. Many cultures used this stone as a protection from evil spirits, deceit, and conspiracy.

In India and other Eastern countries, cat's-eye is worn to correct ill aspects of the South Node of the Moon. In the Orient this stone is said to guard against poverty and evil spirits, while maintaining the good health of the wearer. If pressed to the third eye, cat's-eye is believed to give foresight.

This stone is under the sign of Pisces.

To dream of chrysoberyl cat's-eye is a warning against treachery and waste.

▶ **Healing Energies:** A healing stone for the whole body.

▶ **Magical Powers:** Said to guard the wealth you have and increase it. Prevents financial ruin and will even return what was lost.

MAGICAL USES

To increase your monetary supply, and keep what you have from disappearing on unexpected bills and expenditures, put a cat's-eye into a small green bag with the largest denomination of paper money that you can. Hang this bag over the head of your bed by tacking it to the wall, if necessary. This will be a subconscious reminder every night that you are working to attract prosperity.

Chalcedony

▶ **HARDNESS:** 7

▶ **COLORS:** Many colors.

▶ **SOURCES:** In many places, but primarily mined in Germany, Uruguay, and Brazil.

▶ **FACTS:** A type of microcrystalline quartz, which includes agate, jasper, carnelian, plasma, flint, and chrysoprase, chalcedony develops in cracks and cavities of rocks that are filled by Nature with quartz-rich water. This produces a translucent, waxy stone of white, pale gray, light brown, or bluish color. An outer layer of agate often surrounds chalcedony. In ancient times, its value was quite high. Chalcedony is primarily mined in Brazil and Uruguay.

Some dealers will create imitation sard by saturating chalcedony with an iron solution.

▶ **HISTORY AND FOLKLORE:** The name chalcedony may come from one of the ancient places where it was mined—Chalcedon or Calchedon, an ancient seaport on the Sea of Marmara in Asia Minor. Another possible source for the word chalcedony is from the Greek word *khalkedon* and the Latin *charchedonia*.

The Roman writer Pliny noted that, when heated and rubbed, this stone would attract straw, as does amber. Chalcedony, under the name of *leucachate*, was considered sacred to the goddess Diana.

The Rosicrucians called this stone the "mother stone," and used it to symbolize enthusiasm and divine victory.

In several ancient cultures it was believed that chalcedony protected the traveler on ocean voyages, drove away evil spirits, helped to gain public favor, repelled depression and sadness, and protected the wearer during political revolutions.

At one time, chalcedony was used medicinally for fevers and for the expulsion of gallstones. It was also believed to protect from the evil eye, which was often said to be the underlying cause of illnesses.

Chalcedony is associated with the signs of Cancer and Aquarius, while others say it is associated with Saturn.

To dream of chalcedony means reuniting with lost friends.

▶ **HEALING ENERGIES:** Long used to treat fever, gallstones, and mental problems. Also considered important in increasing lactation of nursing mothers.

▶ **MAGICAL POWERS:** Drives away nightmares, aids in overcoming lawsuits, and repels illusions. Chalcedony can repel any negative incoming vibrations and absorb only positive ones. It also repels bad dreams and night fears.

Brings good fortune. Also aids in creating coherent thoughts.

Blue, gray, purple: helps one get rid of unwanted things in one's life; aids in avoiding messy emotional involvements that will cause distress.

Green: focuses attention on how to relate to others in a loving manner.

Pink: strengthens self-esteem; makes one more aware of and caring about the personal appearance.

White: called the "mother stone." This color of chalcedony shields from negativity, as well as cleanses it out of the aura. Can stabilize the emotions during trying times.

MAGICAL USES

Hang a piece of chalcedony in your car to help prevent accidents. It will also protect you when carried or worn during travel.

Use a piece of white chalcedony to pass over the aura. This will help clean it of any small negative particles that have attached themselves.

Chrysocolla

▶ **HARDNESS:** 2

▶ **COLORS:** Blue-green, bright green, sky blue, or turquoise blue.

▶ **SOURCES:** Found primarily in copper areas in Chile, Russia, and Zaire.

▶ **FACTS:** Chrysocolla usually appears as a crust or in grape-like clusters. Its microcrystalline crystals are often intergrown with quartz, opal, malachite, or turquoise. It is a very soft and light stone, with a texture like enamel. When intergrown with malachite and turquoise, it is known as Eilat Stone,[13] a gem associated with King Solomon's Mines. When mingled with quartz, it is sold under the name of Stellarite; this is different from another stone that uses the same name and is a zoisite.

▶ **HISTORY AND FOLKLORE:** This stone takes its name from the Greek words *chrysos* ("golden") and *kolla* ("cement").

Because it was used as a musical amulet, to dream of chrysocolla was considered very fortunate for musicians, singers, and florists. For centuries, musicians have used this stone as an amulet for healing the throat and lungs.

It is under the sign of Taurus and sometimes associated with Uranus.

To dream of chrysocolla is a sign of unresolved guilt or fear.

▶ **HEALING ENERGIES:** Helps with digestive troubles, high blood pressure, arthritis, and ulcers. Raises the metabolism. Works very well on female problems. Excellent for preventing miscarriage or healing following abortion or hysterectomy.

▶ **MAGICAL POWERS:** Chrysocolla helps to clear the subconscious of fears, guilt, and tension.[14] Aids in releasing old resentments and forgiving people. Helps to calm the emotions. Also good for dealing with the anger and pain of rape or abuse of any kind. A stone with very feminine energies, chrysocolla eases the mental and emotional pains of troubled relationships by relieving tension and bringing out inner strengths.

By working on the throat chakra, it enhances creativity and

communication. Works well in removing blocks to creative energies, whatever the profession.

Makes a bridge of energy between the Earth and sky, the physical and the spiritual planes.

MAGICAL USES

When trying to remove yourself from a troublesome or even dangerous situation or relationship, especially one that is filled with emotional tension, draw a nine-inch circle on a sheet of paper. Set a piece of chrysocolla in the center of the circle. Sit and meditate on what this troubled relationship or situation is costing you in self-esteem, physical danger, mental and emotional stress, even money; make yourself see it in all its ugliness. Do this for nine nights, each time moving the stone a little closer to the edge of the circle. In the meantime, take whatever appropriate and necessary physical action is needed. By the ninth night, you should be able to remove the stone completely from the circle. If, however, you have procrastinated and taken no physical action to help yourself, moving the stone over the edge of the circle will not gain you your freedom from the problem.

Chrysoprase

▶ **HARDNESS:** 7

▶ **COLOR:** A translucent apple green; the green color of this stone comes from nickel.

▶ **SOURCES:** At one time mines in Poland and Czechoslovakia offered the very finest quality of this stone. After 1965, however, the better stones were found in Australia, Brazil, California, the Ural Mountains in Russia, and Austria.

▶ **FACTS:** A variety of quartz chalcedony. If exposed for periods of time to sunlight, this stone's green color will fade to that of jade. This stone has been called the "Mother of Emerald."

▶ **HISTORY AND FOLKLORE:** The name chrysoprase comes from the Greek words *chrysos* ("golden") and *prason* ("a leek"). The ancient Egyptians, Greeks, and Romans held this stone in the highest esteem as the perfect dream stone. Alexander the Great was said to wear a chrysoprase in his girdle or belt at all times. The Egyptians set this stone in rings with lapis lazuli. The Greeks and Romans used it in signet rings and cameos.

Chrysoprase was introduced into England during the reign of Queen Anne; it was her favorite jewel. Later, during the Middle Ages, it was believed that if a condemned person held a chrysoprase in his/her mouth, he/she would become invisible and be able to escape. It remained popular through the reigns of the three King Georges and Queen Victoria.

Chrysoprase was credited with a number of powers: banishing greed, selfishness, and carelessness; stirring the imagination; calming irritability and the pains of gout. It was also said to create happiness, enterprise, prudence, adaptability, versatility, action, progress, and adventure; protect from evil dreams and demons; bring success in new enterprises; and make the wearer cheerful. An old Rumanian legend says that the owner of a chrysoprase will be able to understand the language of lizards.

At one time chrysoprase was believed to hold the Sacred Flame of the Goddess.

It was used in a medicinal way to strengthen the eyes; this could occur only when gazing at this stone when the Moon was passing through Taurus and Cancer.

Chrysoprase is said to be under the sign of Cancer.

To dream of this stone is a warning not to do anything that will draw unwanted attention to yourself.

▶ **HEALING ENERGIES:** A calming, balancing, and healing stone affecting all the bodies, it eases depression and sexual imbalances. Works best on the three upper chakras. Also works on rheumatism and gout.

▶ **MAGICAL POWERS:** It can break neurotic patterns and help one to see the truth in personal problems. Its vibrations have a tranquilizing effect that seems to bring damaging subconscious thoughts to the foreground, where they can be assessed and dealt with. This stone is an aid for balancing attitudes and action, as well as clarifying personal problems and getting to the truth behind them.

This stone can also bring out hidden talents. Gives victory; makes the wearer invisible. Especially inspiring to artists and craftsmen.

MAGICAL USES

Carry or wear this stone to attract prosperity. It also will do double duty as a protector against negative thoughts from other people. Keep chrysoprase on your desk or somewhere in your working area for inspiration and innovative ideas.

Chrysoprase also makes a great altar decoration when worshipping the Goddess.

Cinnabar

▶ **HARDNESS:** 2–2.5
▶ **COLORS:** Reddish brown, orange-red.
▶ **SOURCES:** Spain, Italy, and China.
▶ **FACTS:** Cinnabar, or mercury sulfide, is a brilliant vermilion red color. Its name comes from the Persian word for "dragon's blood,"[15] and is the main ore of mercury. It forms around volcanic vents and hot springs, sometimes in mineral veins. At one time, cinnabar was the main ingredient in vermilion paint, which was first made and used in ancient China. Do not ingest any part of this stone, because it contains poisonous mercury!
▶ **HISTORY AND FOLKLORE:** As far back as 3,600 years ago, the Chinese apothecaries were making and dispensing "pills of immortality" made of cinnabar. How one could have extended life by taking mercury substances is a puzzle.

Cinnabar is often associated with the sign of Gemini.

To dream of this stone indicates a poisonous situation in your life that needs to be dealt with.
▶ **HEALING ENERGIES:** Unknown.
▶ **MAGICAL POWERS:** Helps in becoming dynamic, assertive, and adventurous. Cinnabar is also helpful when you are taking back your personal power after a devastating experience.

MAGICAL USES

Use cinnabar to speed up candle-burning ritual results when you are spelling for the removal of harmful elements in your life. Place the stone between two black candles, with a magenta candle directly behind the stone. Be absolutely certain you are willing to do whatever is necessary to be rid of the people or problems before using this spell.

Citrine

▶ **HARDNESS:** 7

▶ **COLORS:** A clear, pale yellow or golden yellow.

▶ **SOURCES:** Brazil, Spain, Madagascar, and Russia yield the best stones.

▶ **FACTS:** A variety of quartz, whose coloration is due to the presence of iron. Gem-quality citrine of natural color is rare. Much of the citrine on the market is heat-treated amethyst. Although citrine has a good luster and is transparent, its value is quite low in comparison to amethyst and other forms of crystal. It is found in Brazil, North Carolina, California, Spain, and Russia.

At one time, citrine was deliberately marketed under the names of Brazilian topaz, Spanish topaz, and Occidental topaz, in order to fetch the price of topaz, which was considered more valuable at that time.

▶ **HISTORY AND FOLKLORE:** Although citrine was not as popular as other gemstones among ancient cultures, it was used during the Hellenistic Age (323-280 B.C.E.) in Greece. It remained fairly popular for jewelry into the first and second centuries in both Greece and Rome. The name probably is derived from the French word *citron* ("lemon"), referring to its yellow color.

Citrine was at one time used as a talisman against alcoholism, evil thoughts, overindulgences of all kinds, scandal, libel, and treachery.

Medicinally, it was carried as protection against plagues, epidemics, and venomous snake and reptile bites.

Citrine is under the sign of Scorpio.

To dream of citrine is a warning that self-destructive tendencies or attitudes are preventing you from facing and releasing negative karma.

▶ **HEALING ENERGIES:** Found in double terminated, single points, and clusters, citrine's color can range from a yellowish gold to a light brown. It reduces flare-ups from ulcers and helps with digestion. Good for tissue regeneration and detoxifying all the bodies. Works on the circulation, kidneys, heart, gallbladder, liver, and intestines.

▶ **MAGICAL POWERS:** Can eliminate self-destructive tendencies and raise the self-esteem. Use this stone to align with the Higher Self. Related to the navel, or third chakra, citrine can be used to strengthen your self-esteem and protect your aura. It also transforms emotional fears, even inherited ones, by giving clarity of thought.

Aids in working with difficult karma. Its vibrations build up physical, mental, emotional, and spiritual stamina, thus making it possible to positively deal with karmic events. Helps in opening channels to the intuitive levels of the mind.

Known as the abundance stone, citrine attracts prosperity on all levels and is especially good for business success. Increases a person's motivation, and helps in using creative energy. Excellent for those in education and business.

The lighter the color of the citrine, the milder the effect. Use it in combination with aquamarine, blue topaz, or peridot to make one's growth of power and self-control predictable.

MAGICAL USES

A member of the quartz crystal family, citrine can be used in the same way as clear quartz can. The only difference is that its golden yellow color adds Sun energy to the work. When worn, its vibrant shades help to lift the spirits if one is dealing with mild depression or simply feeling down at the time.

This is a very good stone for scrying into matters pertaining to money and other forms of prosperity.

Coral

▶ **HARDNESS:** 3.5–4

▶ **COLORS:** The usual varieties are from the flesh-toned pink through the spectrum to red; also white, blue, gold, and black.

▶ **SOURCES:** Most high-quality coral is fished from the waters of the western Mediterranean Sea, but it is also dredged along the coasts of Greece, the Greek Islands, the Canary Islands, Tunisia, Morocco, Algeria, the Malaysian Archipelago, Japan, Northern Australia, and in the Red Sea. Also found in the Philippines, Hawaii, Indian Ocean, and Alaska.

▶ **FACTS:** Coral is actually an organic material that has solidified into a stone-like substance. It has been used in magic and jewelry for centuries. Coral is formed out of an aggregate of coral polyp skeletons. When alive, these polyps are minute living creatures that live in great colonies. When they die, their remains (mostly calcium carbonate) build up to form coral reefs. The most valuable variety is the branch-like coral called *Corallium rubrum, Corralium Nobile,* or "precious coral."

A special type of black coral (*Antipathes Spiralis*) is harvested from the sea off Hawaii. The Indian Ocean is another source of black coral. Unlike other corals, black coral is composed of an organic material called chitin, which is related to human hair and nails and sheep's wool.

A blue variety (*Allopara subirolcea*) is found around the Philippines and the Cameroons. The coasts of Hawaii, Alaska, Japan, and Australia have an attractive golden coral (*Parazoanthus Spirals*). Fossil coral (*Thamnopora Cevicornis*) is found embedded in limestone deposits and has flower-like markings.

The color-groupings for coral are: Arciscuro, a very dark red, often called ox blood; Rosso Scuro, dark red; Rosso, red; Secondo Coloro, salmon; Rosa Vivo, bright rose; Rosa Pallido, pale rose; and Pelle D'Angello, flesh pink, often called angel skin. The flesh pink coral is usually the most expensive.

The famous Petoskey stones of Lake Michigan are actually fossilized coral.[16]

▶ **HISTORY AND FOLKLORE:** The name coral comes from the Greek word *korallion* and the Latin *corallium*. However, another ancient name, *Gorgeia*, connects it to the Gorgon (Medusa)[17] and the legend of her death at the hands of Perseus. After her death, Perseus put her severed head in a bag and started his long journey home. As he rested beside the sea, he put the sack on a bed of seaweed and brushwood along the edge of the waves. Medusa's blood and power leaked through the weave of the bag and turned the seaweed and brushwood into stone. Sea nymphs came and carried the changed wood and weed to the ocean floor where it became the first coral beds. For this reason, Greeks called red coral Medusa's blood and the ocean's Tree of Life.

Archaeologists have dated the earliest findings of human-used red coral, found in Mesopotamia, at about 3,000 B.C.E.

The most important use of coral by ancient peoples was for protection, particularly against the evil eye. In some cultures still today coral rattles in bells, or simply pieces of coral, are hung in the house to drive away evil spirits. Even the scientist Paracelcus (1495–1541) wrote that evil spirits feared red coral. However, he also warned that such spirits were attracted to brown coral. Part of this belief still remains in the East where to wear dull, discolored, or dirty coral is considered to attract misfortune of all kinds. Other writers say that using brown coral can lead one into the dark side of magic.

From Naples to the south, red coral is still known as "Witch Stone," and is believed to protect against evil magic and bewitchment. Today it is quite common to see little coral hands (closed fist with the index and little finger extended) for sale in jewelry shops, even the expensive ones, as protection against the evil eye.

Another Italian belief is that coral should be hung in the house to repel envy, disharmony, and evil influences. It will also keep away wild animals, prevent nightmares, and protect against lightning. Ancient Greeks fastened red coral to the ship's bows to guide them safely home; it is still common to see coral nailed to the mast of small Mediterranean vessels.

The Romans tied pieces of red coral to cradles and hung coral around the necks of children to ward off disease and help with teething. Coral was also said to prevent epilepsy. Coral jewelry was said to turn pale when the wearer became sick and recover its color when health was restored.

Around the Mediterranean, coral was also attached to fruit and olive trees to ensure a good crop, while women wore it to become pregnant.

Red coral was considered by the Pueblo Indians to be one of the stones of the four elements. Among the Hopi and Zuni, the Road of Life is symbolized by coral, jet, abalone, and turquoise.

In 1564, powdered coral was still being prescribed by physicians for heart problems, hemorrhages, and contagious infections. Coral was hung around the abdomen as a treatment for colic and cramp. In Asia, children had to swallow tiny pieces mixed with plantain for itches. Even in the seventeenth century, coral twigs were boiled in wax and used for urinary problems.

Good pieces of coral are valued as good luck charms for dancers.

To dream of red or pink coral foretells recovery from illness.

Coral is a stone of Venus and under the sign of Pisces.

▶ **HEALING ENERGIES:** The red or white varieties have long been considered helpful in healing mental diseases. Coral is also considered to be helpful for anemia.

▶ **MAGICAL POWERS:** Coral is said to be very useful in rituals to stop or prevent whirlwinds and storms.

By calming the emotions, coral can help with communications and understanding. Repels negative thoughts of ill-wishers.

Blue: helps one to let out the inner child for play.

Black: heals fears and anxieties; good for past life reviews; creates harmony and balance.

Red or white calms storms, gives wisdom, and helps one to cross rivers safely. Also creates emotional openness, affection, and love. As a symbol of life energy, red coral can help you remember what you see and hear during meditation.

Sponge: for a childlike fun mood.

MAGICAL USES

It is possible today to purchase beautiful Southwestern jewelry containing both turquoise and red coral. This can be found in rings, watches, bracelets, and earrings. This type of jewelry not only makes a nice fashion statement, but also is extremely protective in its vibrations.

Hang a piece of red or white coral in your car to help prevent accidents and in your home to protect your possessions, pets, and family. Tuck some in your suitcase when traveling to keep the baggage from getting lost.

Crocidolite (Quartz Cat's-Eye)

▶ **HARDNESS:** 7

▶ **COLORS:** Quartz cat's-eye stones have the usual background color of greenish gray, golden yellow, or green; the fibrous inclusions produce the chatoyancy, or eye, when properly cut, usually in a cabochon form. On very rare occasions, however, cat's-eye quartz can be hyacinth red, greenish yellow, or gray. The bull's-eye (sometimes called the ox-eye) is a mahogany color.

▶ **SOURCES:** Cat's-eye stones come mostly from Sri Lanka, West Germany, and Burma. Hawk's-eye, bull's-eye, and the plentiful tiger's-eye come primarily from South Africa.

▶ **FACTS:** Quartz eye stones with the names of cat's-eye, tiger's-eye, hawk's-eye, and bull's-eye are technically called crocidolite. When cut *en cabochon*, these quartz stones produce an eye-like effect when light moves over them. This is known as chatoyancy, and is caused by fibrous inclusions within the stones. (See separate entries under Hawk's-Eye and Tiger's-Eye.)

▶ **HISTORY AND FOLKLORE:** The Arabs said this stone could make the wearer invisible in battle. It was also used to protect against dark sorcery and death. The ancient Assyrians put all kinds of cat's-eye stones in statues of their deities; they greatly valued this stone as a charm against sorcery.

In India, the cat's-eye is one of the Nine Sacred Gems and greatly valued. It is said that this stone draws wealth and keeps it from being lost. It is also powerful against nightmares and for success in speculation and games of chance. In India and other Eastern countries, cat's-eye is worn to correct ill aspects of the South Node of the Moon. Cat's-eye gives mental balance, foresight, and attractiveness.

In medicine, this stone was used to relieve depression, cure chronic disorders, and put color in pale faces. When used as a birth charm, it was wrapped with a female hair of a woman who had already successfully, and easily, given birth. Cat's-eye rubbed on the eyelids was thought to relieve inflammation.

Cat's-eye is believed to help with the thinking processes and will aid with foresight if it is pressed against the third eye. It was worn as a success charm when engaging in speculative business ventures, as cat's-eye was said to prevent financial distress and ruin.

Cat's-eye was associated with the signs of Leo and Capricorn.

Traditionally, to dream of cat's-eye warns to be watchful for treachery through business acquaintances or friends. It can also mean to be watchful for coming opportunities.

► **HEALING ENERGIES:** Wear to aid the stomach and digestion. It is never advisable to swallow a stone, even if the stone is not poisonous.

► **MAGICAL POWERS:** A charm against evil spirits, this stone attracts the gift of foresight and intensifies psychic awareness. Will bring wealth and prevent its loss. Can be a dangerous stone if used only to gratify the ego; for example, someone who is miserly will find the wealth constantly trickling away instead of amassing.

MAGICAL USES

Personally, I like quartz cat's-eye, or crocidolite, better than I like the chrysoberyl cat's-eye. Often you cannot see much difference between the two kinds of stones, except the exorbitant price charged for the chrysoberyl.

Wear cat's-eye to be alert to everything that is going on around you.

Since this stone also activates your psychic awareness, this alertness will include intuitive messages and warnings. This is especially valuable when you are in a tense situation and might need to make split second decisions, moving into action immediately. This alertness is also handy in any competitive situation where quick thinking might mean much in the way of career advancement or getting a good deal on something.

Danburite

- ► **HARDNESS:** 7
- ► **COLORS:** Colorless, wine yellow, pink, sometimes streaked with white.
- ► **SOURCES:** Connecticut, Myanmar, Mexico, Switzerland, Italy, and Japan.
- ► **FACTS:** Danburite forms in wedge-shaped prisms, similar to colorless topaz, but has poor cleavage. It was first found in Danbury, Connecticut, from which it took its name. Although the faceted stones are bright, they lack fire. Large clear crystals are rare.
- ► **HISTORY AND FOLKLORE:** None known.

    A little-known stone that is not in many collections, danburite is associated with Aries.

    To dream of this stone means beware of hasty words that will come back to haunt you later.
- ► **HEALING ENERGIES:** Unknown.
- ► **MAGICAL POWERS:** Excellent for impatient people, particularly those who lose control in a slow line at the counter or in a traffic jam.

MAGICAL USES

If you are an extremely impatient person who easily loses her/his cool, and possibly temper as well, try meditating frequently while holding danburite. You can also carry danburite with you and use it as a worry stone to remind yourself to be more patient and understanding of situations that are out of your control.

Diamond

▶ **HARDNESS:** 10

▶ **COLORS:** Colorless, steel, pink, blue, green, canary yellow, orange, green, cinnamon, and black.

▶ **SOURCES:** Today, diamonds are taken from sources in Siberia, Africa, India, Brazil, Ghana, Sierra Leone, Zaire, Botswana, Namibia, and the U.S., with Australia being the main producer.

▶ **FACTS:** Diamond is the hardest natural stone on Earth, being nearly 150 times harder than corundum which is the second hardest; the hardness of all other gems and stones is measured against that of the diamond. Made of carbon atoms, diamonds were formed in magma chambers deep in the Earth; sometimes these veins, or pipelines as they are called, were thousands of meters in height. The usual natural form of a diamond is octahedral (two four-sided pyramids, base to base), although some are dodecahedrons (12 lozenge-shaped faces) or icositetrahedrons (24 kite-shaped faces). They are sorted into five grades, the lowest being indus-trial. Although commonly known as clear, diamonds can come in a variety of colors, such as pink, blue, green, canary yellow, cinna-mon, and black. In certain parts of Asia, the blood red diamond, or a diamond spotted with red, was considered to bring disaster to any owner.

Until the eighteenth century, most diamonds came from India, where they were mined along with gold, ruby, sapphire, and garnet from alluvial deposits. India traded diamonds around the Middle East as early as 800 B.C.E.. The first diamonds brought to Europe arrived in 1584 from Sumbulpour, India, the first known mine of the Golconda kingdom. The diamond mines of Brazil began excavating this stone in 1728. Finally, diamonds were dis-covered in 1851 in New South Wales, Australia, and first dug on a large, commercial scale near Kimberley, South Africa, in 1867.

▶ **HISTORY AND FOLKLORE:** Some writers believe that the name dia-mond came from the Greek words *adamas, adamantos,* which mean "adamant." However, Hindu writers of an earlier period link the stone with the Sanskrit word *dyu*, "a deity." The Eastern goddess Dia is still called the Diamond Sow, and her yonic shrine in paradise is known as the Diamond Seat.

In ancient times, only members of royal families were allowed to wear diamonds. However, the Persians thought that this stone was sinful because the devil had created it. Other cultures, including India, believed that diamonds were created when thunderbolts struck the Earth.

The Romans wore a diamond on the left arm for victory over one's enemies and to gain bravery. If it were set in steel, it was thought to prevent insanity. Also known as the Stone of Reconciliation, the diamond was said to repel all sorcery and nightmares, as well as strengthen friendships. The Greeks called this stone the Holy Necessity, emblem of the Sun.

The Hebrews considered the diamond to be the most powerful of all the gems, even overshadowing the mystical, forceful lodestone.

During the Middle Ages, knights set diamonds in their armor, shields, and sword hilts as talismans for protection and victory. These diamonds were mounted in their rough form as the ability to facet diamonds was yet unknown. By the thirteenth century in Italy, the diamond was known as *amante di Dio* ("lover of God") and was widely considered a sacred stone for religious purposes. When Vasco de Gama discovered a new sea route to India, the trade in diamonds increased.

This gemstone did not become accessible or "fashionable" to the middle classes until Agnes Sorel, mistress of Charles VII of France, was given a diamond and gold necklace by the wealthy merchant, Jacques Coeur.

When Elizabeth I ruled England, it became a fad to wear "scribbling rings," which were made by inserting a diamond octahedron into a heavy gold ring. The young dandies would use the sharp point of the diamond to scratch poetry on the windows of whichever lady caught their eyes.

During the 1600s, the French explorer J. B. Tavernier traveled to the Far East where he personally saw the great Peacock Throne in Delhi. He described this Throne as having a canopy whose underside was covered with pearls and diamonds. On the top a Peacock stood with a spread-tail of sapphires and other stones, while hanging before the king's eye was a diamond pendant of about 80–90 carats. On each side of the Throne were two parasols with diamond-covered handles.

According to Al Kazwani, an Arabian philosopher of the ninth century, Alexander the Great discovered a valley of diamonds near the land of "Hind." However, this valley was guarded by serpents that killed by their gaze. In *A Thousand and One Nights*, a collection of tales told by Scheherazade, concubine of a powerful Arabian king, there is a story of Sinbad who also found a valley of diamonds guarded by poisonous snakes. A similar story is found in the writings of Marco Polo; he said the valley was in the kingdom of "Motupali," which has now been established as Golconda, in Hyderabad.

The ancient Persians and Arabs believed that the diamond brought great good fortune; this belief is still held by modern Egyptians. Writing in the fourteenth century C.E., the mystic Rabbi Benoni said that the diamond was so powerful that it could produce a state of ecstasy, protect against evil, and attract planetary influences. However, Sir John Mandeville, an English traveler of the fourteenth century, wrote that he knew it to be possible for a diamond to lose its positive virtues if handled by evil people.

Powdered diamonds have been used in medicine and magic by a number of cultures. Hindu physicians used diamond powder to ensure strength, energy, beauty, clear skin, happiness, and long life; however, the powder had to come from flawless diamonds. In Spain diamond dust was a common ingredient in medicine to treat the plague and bladder diseases. As late as 1532, physicians were prescribing diamond powder, along with other precious stones, for Pope Clement VII.

The diamond, of all gemstones, has perhaps the most evil-fated legends attached to some of its largest specimens. The malevolency of large diamonds was known far back in ancient history. The cultures that were familiar with the diamond said the large stones should never be worn as ornaments. To do so would bring disaster, misfortune, and sudden death. In fact, diamonds were considered an unlucky stone by some people (mostly Europeans) well into the sixteenth century. To lose any diamond was considered a dread omen of misfortune to come. However, in both India and ancient Rome, the diamond as a whole was thought to be extremely lucky. The malevolency may have arisen from strong negative thoughts of someone who handled a particular diamond and imprinted it with these thoughts.

The Koh-I-Noor ("Mountain of Light"), which is now set in one of the British crowns, originally came from India and has a male misfortune attached to it. No male British sovereign is ever allowed to wear the crown containing this diamond. Before England possessed this Indian diamond, however, it was frequently dipped in water to heal every kind of sickness.

The Sancy diamond, weighing 55 carats, was purchased in Turkey about 1570 by the Seigneur de Sancy from France. It was loaned by him to Henry III, but the messenger who carried the stone was horribly murdered. The recovered stone was years later sold to the Astor family.

The Regent diamond, now on display in the Louvre, was found in 1701 by an Indian slave on the River Kistna in India. It weighs 410 carats. The slave managed to escape with the diamond, but was murdered by the captain of the ship on which he sailed. The captain later hanged himself. The diamond was later purchased by the William Pitt family of Britain. They had the stone cut into a 140 carat cushion shape. The Duke of Orleans purchased the faceted diamond in 1717. In 1722 Louis XIV set it into his crown, and Napoleon even used it as a decoration on his coronation sword.

The Florentine (a citron yellow) was owned by Charles the Bold, Duke of Burgundy, and also by the powerful Medici family. After being lost on a battlefield in 1477, it was seen by the French explorer Tavernier in the treasury of the Grand Duke of Tuscany. Later it came to the Hapsburgs through the marriage of the Duke of Tuscany to Empress Marie Theresa of Austria. When the royal family went into exile in Switzerland, the diamond was stolen and sold in South America. The Florentine was said to be cut as a double rose with nine irregular sides; it weighed 137.27 carats.

In 1668, King Louis XIV bought a blue diamond weighing 112 carats, which became known as "The Blue Diamond of the Crown." The king ordered it recut, reducing its weight to 67.50 carats. It was stolen during the French Revolution and disappeared. However, some experts believe that the Hope diamond is actually this lost blue gemstone.

The Hope got its name from one of its owners, Henry Phillip Hope, a banker and gem collector. He purchased the stone in 1830 for $90,000. It is at this point that the bad luck stories began to accumulate around this particular diamond. When Hope's nephew inherited the stone, he soon lost his fortune. A Turkish sultan who purchased it in 1908 lost his Sultanate and nearly his life in a revolution. He sold it to Mrs. Edward McLean, wife of the owner of the *Washington Post* in 1911. Although she lost her personal fortune and her son to an accident, she refused to believe in the diamond's bad luck reputation.

Originally, the diamond was said to protect its owner from the plague and ward off evil spirits. It was this belief that led, in the sixteenth century, to the giving of diamonds in rings as tokens of affection. The diamond is believed to drive away evil dreams, render poisons harmless, prevent enchantment, and repel wild beasts, demons, and evil men. Its bad luck reputation may come from a logical source: the imprinting of a particular stone with negative vibrations from people who touch it or strong emotional events that happen around it.

This stone is connected with Aries, the Sun, and Spring.

To dream of diamonds symbolizes victory over enemies. It can also mean the satisfactory completion of any venture.

▶ **HEALING ENERGIES:** Known as a Master Healer, this stone breaks up blockages in both the crown chakra and in the personality.

▶ **MAGICAL POWERS:** Diamond is considered to be a magical stone of great power. It enhances all energies in the body, mind, and spirit, thus helping with alignment with the Higher Self. It also helps with all functions of the brain, and gives victory, great strength, and courage.

MAGICAL USES

The average person is not going to be able to purchase a diamond of any size to use in magical work. However, small diamond chips set in jewelry can be affordable if you shop around. Regardless of some of the written work that emphatically states only loose stones will work, being in a setting does not impede the diamond's energy in any way, and often intensifies it instead.

When in a relaxed mood, turn the jewelry slowly in a low-level light or candlelight until you get flashes from the diamond. Oftentimes, when in a pensive frame of mind, this in itself will open the door to the subconscious mind and allow intuitive messages to slip through. The flashes can also set off bits of past-life memories, information that can help you to understand a particular present-day problem.

Diopside

▶ **HARDNESS:** 5.5

▶ **COLORS:** Usually bottle green, brownish green, or light green, but may be colorless, white, brown, black, or violet.

▶ **SOURCES:** Myanmar, Siberia, Pakistan, South Africa, Austria, Brazil, Italy, the U.S., Madagascar, Canada, India, and Sri Lanka.

▶ **FACTS:** The more iron-rich diopside is, the darker the green, sometimes being almost black. The very bright green crystals are colored by chromium, while the violet ones are colored by manganese. Since 1964, dark green and black diopside has been found in southern India; this is cut *en cabochon* to produce a four-rayed star. Star stones have always been thought to have a helpful spirit inside them. Some even display chatoyancy, or the cat's-eye effect.

The violet blue crystals, also called violane, have been found in Italy and the U.S. If violane is massive, it is ordinarily cut in beads. When transparent and fibrous, it is cut *en cabochon* for collectors.

A plain green variety of diopside is found in the Ala Valley in Italy; this is called alalite.[18]

▶ **HISTORY AND FOLKLORE:** None known.

Diopside is often associated with the planet Jupiter.

To dream of diopside symbolizes a need to rethink plans and goals.

▶ **HEALING ENERGIES:** This stone is said to reduce fevers and body aches.

▶ **MAGICAL POWERS:** Aids in making connections with spiritual teachers and guides.

MAGICAL USES

Diopside is a good stone to carry or wear during Jupiter retrogrades. Its gentle but steady vibrations and energies helps to mitigate most negative effects that the retrograde may cause in your personal life.

Dioptase

▶ **HARDNESS:** 5

▶ **COLORS:** Usually a beautiful, vivid emerald green; can be blue-green.

▶ **SOURCES:** Russia, Namibia, Zaire, Chile, and Arizona.

▶ **FACTS:** Sometimes confused with dark emerald, dioptase has a hint of blue in it. This stone has a high fire that is undetectable because of its deep rich coloring; the stones tend to be translucent. Too brittle and fragile to be worn, dioptase is cut for the collector. Sometimes specimens of matrix rock with veins or crusts of dioptase are offered for sale. Another name for this stone is sometimes given as "copper emerald."

▶ **HISTORY AND FOLKLORE:** None known.

Dioptase is sometimes connected with Venus.

To dream of this stone means more thought and planning need to go into your life.

▶ **HEALING ENERGIES:** Healing for any problem or disease with the brain.

▶ **MAGICAL POWERS:** A new stone to the magical world, dioptase appears to work well in the fields of plant growth, getting pregnant, or getting in touch with Nature spirits.

MAGICAL USES

To heal unhealthy plants, you really need to get in touch with the Nature spirits that are responsible for them. Place a piece of dioptase in the pot, or near the base of the plant with the problems. Ask the plant spirits to accept the stone as payment for helping you heal the plant. Talk to both the plant and the Nature spirits, encouraging them to produce healthier growth. Leave the stone there, even after the plant recovers.

Emerald

▶ **HARDNESS:** 7.5–8
▶ **COLORS:** Shades of green, with dark emerald green being the most sought after. Those found in the old Cleopatra mines are a lighter color.
▶ **SOURCES:** Colombia, other South American countries.
▶ **FACTS:** A variety of beryl colored by chromium whose crystals are hexagonal in shape. It is far more difficult to find a top-quality emerald than it is to find such a gemstone of others in the beryl family. Rarely found as clean crystals, most emeralds are heavily flawed with inclusions. These inclusions are called *jardin* ("garden"), because they resemble leaves and branches. However, these inclusions are like a fingerprint, enabling you to tell the difference between a natural and laboratory emerald, and to separate one natural emerald from another. Emerald is one of the few gemstones that can contain deep flaws and still command a high price.

One strange fact is that emeralds will "sweat" when subjected to heat; that is, they will lose water. Ancient writings speak of this phenomenon.

The Chivor and Muzo mines of Colombia, South America, produce the biggest and most beautiful emeralds. Smaller quantities of medium-light colored stones are found in Brazil, the Transvaal, Zimbabwe, Zambia, Tanzania, India, Pakistan, the Urals, and Austria. Fine-colored, deep emeralds of more than two carats are very valuable.

There are also golden emeralds, but they are extremely rare.

▶ **HISTORY AND FOLKLORE:** The word emerald could have come from three different root sources: the Greek *smaragdos*, the Latin *smaragdus*, or the old French *esmerald*.

Emeralds were known to the Egyptians and other ancient cultures before 2,000 B.C.E. Most of the emerald mines at that time were in Upper Egypt near the Red Sea. The most famous of these mines was in Mount Zabarah and was said to belong to the Queen of Sheba; the location of this mine was rediscovered in 1818. Legend says that some of the earliest emerald crystals from these mines were so huge (up to twenty feet long) that they were used as temple pillars.[19]

The Egyptian *Book of the Dead* says that the god Thoth gave the emerald to the Egyptians. Embalmers were instructed to place an emerald at the throat of every mummy to give youthful strength and protection during the journey through the Underworld. The god Thoth, master of magic, was said to be the first owner the famous Emerald Tablet of the later magician Hermes Trismegistus; this Tablet was believed to be made of *uat*, or matrix emerald. The god Horus was also connected with the emerald through one of his names: Prince of the Emerald Stone.

Sacred to the Great Goddess, emerald was used in the celebration of many Spring festivals. Because it was called a stone of Venus or Aphrodite, emerald was considered strongest if worn on Her holy day, Friday.[20]

The Etruscans, Phoenicians, and Romans got their emeralds from Habach in the Taurus Mountains. The Romans believed that nothing evil could remain in the presence of an emerald; if powerless to repel misfortune, it was believed the stone would fall from its setting as a warning. The decadent emperor Nero watched the gladiatorial fights through an emerald because he believed the stone not only protected his eyes, but also revealed the truth.

An old belief also says that an emerald will change color if lies and treachery are planned within its vicinity. Many a husband gave his wife an emerald, believing that the stone would shatter if she committed adultery. In India and ancient Egypt, the emerald was said to give the gift of memory, good luck, and reveal ancient secrets and future knowledge.

The emerald had a mystic religious significance to many religions, including Christianity. This stone was often carried or worn as an amulet to focus the mind on spiritual matters. To the Muslims, the emerald represents their first heaven. In India, if one gives an emerald to a deity one could expect to receive the gift of knowledge of the soul and eternal life; they associated the emerald with Taurus. Rosicrucians believe that wearing a gold ring set with an emerald on the solar finger of the left hand will manifest one's deepest desires and wishes. The Christians looked at this stone as the symbol of triumph over sin.

Mystics have long considered the emerald to be of the highest worth among gemstones, because of its strong ability to help with all types of divination, whether of a spiritual or secular nature. If worn during an honest business transaction, the emerald is said to aid the wearer's intuition, thus swinging the transaction in his/her favor.

During the Crusades, the word emerald was used to describe any green gemstone, simply because Europeans did not know the difference in stones. Thus, many stones taken or bought by the Crusaders as "emeralds" were actually chrysolites and peridots.

At one time, during the late 1800s or early 1900s, many of the gems of the Mogul emperors of Delhi were displayed in Europe. One talismanic emerald weighed 78 carats and was a deep rich green. Around its edge were Persian characters declaring that the owner enjoyed the special protection of God.

In the Manta valley in Peru the people were said to have an emerald the size of an ostrich egg, which they called the Goddess Esmeralda. Smaller emeralds, called "daughters," were brought to this goddess' temple as offerings.[21] When the Spanish invaded South America during the sixteenth century, they looted the

Temple of the Sun with its large collection of emeralds, but never found the Temple of Esmeralda. Its location is still a mystery.

As with certain diamonds, there have been specific emeralds that were considered malevolent in nature. Philip II of Spain ruled during the era of the Spanish Armada when a certain circle appeared. This gold ring held an emerald cut to contain a ring of diamonds. The church that received the ring as a gift was completely destroyed by fire. The ring was rescued from the fire and given to a museum, which was soon after struck by lightning and seriously damaged. Those in authority secretly buried the ring in an iron coffin; its resting place is unknown.

Another infamous emerald ring belonged to the Russian royal family. The Empress Elizabeth Petrovna gave this ring to Peter of Holstein-Gottorp, who later became Peter III of Russia. He was assassinated. The Emperor Paul wore it and was strangled to death. Unwilling to dispose of the ring, Alexander II had it reset; it slid off his finger when he was assassinated. Alexander III was smarter than the others; although he kept the ring in the royal treasury, he refused to wear it. However, his son Nicholas II wore it; his entire family was murdered during the Russian Revolution. The whereabouts of the ring is unknown today.

As with other gemstones, the emerald was used for medicinal purposes. In the East, physicians said the emerald cured epilepsy, removed pain, stopped vomiting, was an antidote to stings and bites, remedied jaundice and diabetes, and could cure leprosy if applied as a poultice. As late as the seventeenth century, salts and tinctures of emerald were used to treat dysentery, heart disease, melancholy, and head pains. Doctors also believed that this stone cured inflammation and infections of the eye as well as enhanced the sight. In fact, no pharmacy or alchemist's shop in the Middle Ages would have been without emerald. For centuries engravers kept an emerald at hand to gaze at when their eyes tired.

The emerald has long been connected with the goddess Diana/Artemis, deity of the forest, guardian of women and young girls, and the patroness of childbirth. Thus, emerald talismans came to be worn by women to stop miscarriage and grant an easy birth. This stone was believed to crack if a woman's chastity was violated; thus, it was a favorite stone for husbands to give to wives. Paracelsus wrote that the emerald's vibrations worked best with copper, a metal belonging to Venus.

Ancient astrologers linked this stone to Mercury. The emerald was carried by travelers and sailors as a talisman to ensure a safe journey and bring good fortune, all aspects under Mercury's control.

There were also other uses for an emerald talisman. Parents hung it on their children's necks to protect from leprosy and the plague. Lovers exchanged emeralds, believing that the stone would lose its color should one be unfaithful. The emerald was also used as protection from enchantment, the evil eye, poisonous snakes, epilepsy, hemorrhages, demonic possession, and to exorcise evil spirits.

Emerald is associated with the zodiacal signs of Taurus, Gemini, and Aries.

To dream of an emerald signifies worldly benefit and goodness, a time of happiness where you have much to look forward to.

▶ **HEALING ENERGIES:** A high energy stone, emerald is a valuable healing stone. It strengthens the eyes, heart, immune and nervous systems.

▶ **MAGICAL POWERS:** A tonic for body, mind, and spirit, this stone aids in the alignment of all the bodies. Extremely balancing for one seeking the truth. Said to ward off negativity and strengthen spiritual insight. Helps with and enhances dreams, meditation, and the striving for deeper spiritual insight. Can also foretell the future if used as a scrying stone.

Emerald is said to attract prosperity, peace, balance, love, healing, and patience. Reveals the truth, especially regarding a lover, and protects against all enchantments. Helps with the memory and speech; sharpens the wits. Softens arrogance and balances energies.

Helps one to use creative abilities along with focused organization. Associated with Venus and the Moon, the emerald imparts creativity, strengthens artistic abilities, and opens the way to new beginnings.

It can charge and magnetize other stones or objects with its power, as well as focus this power in a powerful beam.

Some writers say that the week prior to and following a Full Moon is the best time to use an emerald, with the night of the Full Moon being the strongest. It is at these times that the stone's powers are the greatest.

MAGICAL USES

Colombian emeralds are the clearest and most vivid green, and also the most expensive. Other emeralds will be less transparent and the price more reasonable. More expensive, a better green, and less opaqueness does not mean stronger vibrational energies. As with any stone, each emerald must be judged individually for strength.

Many of the old records recommend that an emerald be set in either silver or copper. An emerald set in a sterling silver ring, for example, is an outstanding, eye-catching piece of jewelry without a doubt. The combination of silver and emerald also sensitizes the wearer to intuitive ideas and psychic aid, particularly in the field of the creative arts.

Sleep with an emerald under your pillow to help you remember your dreams and astral travels.

Epidote

▶ **HARDNESS:** 6.5

▶ **COLORS:** Pistachio, yellow green, green, dark brown.

▶ **SOURCES:** Austrian and French Alps, Russia, Italy, island of Elba, and Mozambique, Mexico.

▶ **FACTS:** Infrequently cut as a gemstone, epidote forms in columnar prisms. It is almost equal in hardness to quartz, but its dark color usually makes this stone appear to be opaque. The darkest crystals, which can look as if they are black, can be mistaken for schorl, or black tourmaline. When viewed from different directions, epidote will strongly flash colors of yellow, green, or brown.

Granite rocks containing high percentages of green epidote

and pink feldspar are polished or tumbled and sold as unakite. A rare emerald green variety of this stone found in Burma is sold under the name of tawmawite. Epidote is a member of the zoisite family, along with thulite and tanzanite.

▶ **HISTORY AND FOLKLORE:** None known.

▶ **HEALING ENERGIES:** Unknown.

▶ **MAGICAL POWERS:** Epidote can help you to remain powerful in a situation in which you would usually be victimized. It protects the third chakra, and aids in steady evolution of the self.

MAGICAL USES

Hold epidote to the navel chakra for short periods of time when working to overcome situations that threaten your personal power and well-being. Wear this stone or hold during meditation when searching for answers to emotional situations.

Eye Agate and Fire Agate: see Agate

Flint

▶ **HARDNESS:** 7

▶ **COLORS:** Many colors.

▶ **SOURCE:** Worldwide.

▶ **FACTS:** The name flint is derived from the Greek word *plinthos,* which means a brick. It consists almost entirely of silica with a little lime, oxide of iron, water, carbon, and sometimes traces of organic matter. Classed as a variety of chalcedony, flint can be found in the colors of gray-white, gray, black, light brown, red, and yellow. This stone is usually found in nodular shape with a white crust caused by weathering. Although it is a tough substance, flint can be easily worked. The Neolithic cultures chipped and formed this stone into all kinds of weapons and tools.

▶ **HISTORY AND FOLKLORE:** Flint was one of the first materials used by early humans to make tools and weapons. It chips easily, leaving extremely sharp edges. In ancient Egypt, flint was used to make the first incision in a body prior to embalming.

During the Middle Ages, flint arrowheads were unearthed all over Europe; these were thought to be the fossilized tongues of snakes, on the same order as the fossil teeth of ancient sharks. These, and the flint hammerheads, were mounted in silver as protective amulets, or simply had a hole drilled through them for the same purpose. The arrowheads were thought to prevent bewitchment by elves and fairies and are sometimes called Elf Shot or Fairy Dart. They were also said to be useful in guarding the house against lightning strikes. The hammerheads, connected by the Norse people with the god Thorr, were believed to have the same influence against thunder and lightning. This idea may have been influenced by the fact that flint striking hard metals will produce sparks.

As far back as 300 B.C.E., physicians were crediting flint with the ability to break up kidney and bladder stones, although how it was used for this purpose was not recorded. Pieces of flint with a natural hole through it were said to prevent stomach disorders if worn; if placed under the bed, they relieved cramps and rheumatism. In Scandinavia, midwives poured great quantities of ale through a holed flint to ensure an easy childbirth. However, most of the uses for flint were magical in nature.

In northern England, it is not unusual to find a flint with a natural hole in it hanging in a dairy. It seems that in many European countries this amulet was used to prevent the curdling of milk during thunderstorms and the harassing of the animals by evil spirits, elves, or fairies. Called Hag Stones, Holey Stones, Nightmare or Witch Riding Stones, these holed flints were said to prevent both people and animals from suffering enchantments. Oftentimes, the holed flint was tied around the neck or to the key to the dairy, barn, or stable.

In Ireland, sick people were often treated by giving them a drink made by soaking a flint arrowhead in water for a time. Horses and cattle considered to be wounded by "fairy darts" were given the same treatment.

Any Irish woman during the Middle Ages who found a flint arrowhead or fossil shark's tooth was given the position of village medical counselor. Until quite recently in Ireland, farm workers often wore the *saigead* talismans (a flint arrowhead set in silver) to prevent spells being put on them by the fairies and elves.

In the Scandinavian countries, it was common to find ancient flint knives in the homes. These were treated as holy objects and often "fed" with melted butter and beer.

Flint is associated with the element of Earth.

To dream of flint symbolizes you are not seeing the reality behind an illusion.

▶ **HEALING ENERGIES:** Breaking up and removing kidney and bladder stones. Relieves cramps and rheumatism.

▶ **MAGICAL POWERS:** Helps one to survive no matter what happens. Excellent for survivors who have undergone abuse of any kind or any traumatic event.

MAGICAL USES

Flint can be purchased in any number of forms, from tiny arrowheads to modern-made flint knives. Just remember that the edges can be extremely sharp.

Flint is most useful in getting in touch with the Fairy Folk, Nature spirits, and Earth elementals. It seems to act like a signal that says, "I'm open to acknowledging your existence and would really like to know you better." Put a piece of flint on your altar to attract the help of these Otherworld beings during spellworking and ritual. Use a flint knife in place of a metal athame for casting a magical circle. Meditate with flint nearby, and your contacts with the Fairy Folk and other such beings will be clearer and stronger. Use a piece of flint attached to a chain for pendulum dowsing or just ordinary pendulum work.

Fluorite

▶ **HARDNESS:** 4

▶ **COLORS:** Wide range of colors.

▶ **SOURCES:** Canada, the U.S., South Africa, Thailand, Peru, Mexico, China, Poland, Hungary, Czechoslovakia, Norway, England, Germany, and Switzerland.

▶ **FACTS:** At one time called fluorspar, fluorite is relatively soft. Frequently, there is more than one color in a single stone. The largest crystals have been found in the United States, while expensive pink ones are found in the Alps in Switzerland. England has a purple and yellow banded variety known as Blue John. It is sometimes intergrown with rock quartz crystal. A typical characteristic of fluorite is cubic crystal twins; these are two crystals that are intergrown.

Sometimes fluorite has yellow rutiles running through it.

▶ **HISTORY AND FOLKLORE:** The ancient Egyptians knew of fluorite and carved it into statues and scarabs. The cultures in China have been using fluorite in carvings for over 300 years.

The Roman Augustus Caesar took six fluorite vases from Alexandria, while Pompey raided six such vases from a treasury and presented them to the temple of Jupiter in Rome. Carved fluorite ornaments were recovered from the ruins of Pompeii. Even the historian Pliny knew of fluorite, although he called it *murrhine*.

Physicians during the eighteenth century recommended powdered fluorite in water to relieve kidney disease.

Fluorite is connected with Pisces and Capricorn.

To dream of fluorite means you need to ground and balance yourself if you are to grow spiritually.

▶ **HEALING ENERGIES:** Good for blood vessels and the spleen. Similar to the healing qualities of amethyst.

▶ **MAGICAL POWERS:** Helps to ground excessive energy, particularly mental, emotional, and nervous energy. A powerful healer, it affects all the chakras as well as mental attitudes.

Excellent for cleansing the aura; also rids it of any cording (unwanted attached energy lines from other people). Repels unwanted cordings; to do this, hold to the third eye for about fifteen seconds.

Aids in channeling. Excellent for connecting with the Akashic records for answers to your past lives. Can be used for scrying by holding a rather transparent piece of fluorite in front of a candle. Excellent for concentration and meditation as it enhances the ability to understand more advanced abstract concepts and access past lives. Aids interdimensional communications, particularly with Nature spirits, fairies, elves, and such.

Fluorite is useful in increasing concentration and achieving alignment and harmony with the universe. It also fosters mental balance. Nicknamed the "genius stone," fluorite, singular or in clusters, is excellent for study and work areas. It helps the mind to stay focused on the prime intention.

Fluorite can act as a transformational catalyst, helping to enhance meditation, ground excess energy, and open the higher mind to cosmic wisdom. Use with other stones to amplify their effect.

MAGICAL USES

Keep a piece of fluorite on your desk to help you concentrate when working or studying. Set on your altar or sacred space with other stones to enhance their powers. Hold it while meditating; this will help to still busy thoughts and troublesome emotions that may be bothering you. Store fluorite with your magical tools and jewelry to strengthen their powers. Carry a piece in your car to aid in soothing emotions ruffled during prime-time traffic snarls. Sleep with it under your pillow to help with insomnia and to coax the Fairy Folk to communicate with you during the night.

Fossils

▶ **HARDNESS:** 6–6.5
▶ **COLORS:** Many colors.
▶ **SOURCE:** Worldwide.
▶ **FACTS:** A fossil is described as any plant or animal that existed before the end of the last glacial epoch. The word fossil comes from the Latin *fossilis*, which means something that is dug up. This can include plants, animals, bones, shells, scales, and even pieces of wood. Also in this classification are the imprints of such things as feet, fins, or leaves, in other words, a natural cast of any organism. Eggs and excrement of animals can also become fossilized.

Specialists in the field of paleontology have divided fossils into three categories of studies: vertebrate paleontology, which studies animals with an internal bony skeleton, such as fish, amphibians, reptiles, birds, and mammals; invertebrate paleontology, which studies protozoans, sponges, coral, starfish, shell animals, and insects; and paleobotanists who are concerned only with ancient plant life.

Through millions of years the original bone or shell or fibrous structure is slowly replaced by minerals. The mineral pyrite often replaces bones and shells in fossils, as does opal, calcite, quartz, dolomite, and agate. However, often the original cellular structure can still be seen in minute detail.

One specimen of sea life fossilized in agate is called the turitella; this is a black agate dotted with gray and white little fossils. The turitella, along with the ammonite and others, has a very ancient history of magical use.

Ammonites are spiral-shaped sea creatures that became fossilized. During the Middle Ages, they were called *draconites*, because they were believed to come from the heads of dragons. Another name for this fossil is snakestone; it is famed in occult circles for its magical powers. However, because many people think snake stone is a petrified snake, a lot of snake stone sold today is nothing more than an ammonite that has had a snake's head carved at one end. Actually, this carving does nothing for the fossil except ruin its original beauty.

Copralite is actually petrified dinosaur dung. In fact, the name copralite means "excrement stone." It can be tan, brown, or mottled with red, green, and brown. This can be anywhere from two to two million years old. If cut and polished like agates, copralite shows extraordinarily beautiful colors.

Tigillite is fossilized worm tunnels. It is also possible to find or purchase fossilized sea dollars with their natural five-point star design. Ancient sponges, known as Witch stones," are round and have a natural hole through them.

► **HISTORY AND FOLKLORE:** The ritual use of fossils has a very ancient history. Hundreds of them have been excavated from Neolithic burial sites all over Europe. Shamans around the world still consider fossils valuable tools to amplify magical energy.

Not a gemstone, but a fossil, the ammonite has held an important place in the history of magic and is still used today. It is the fossil of a mollusk (extinct for millions of years) with a flat, spiral-shaped shell, which can reach up to 30 centimeters in diameter. One specimen, now on display at Cardiff Museum in Wales, measures about two meters in diameter. The mollusk shell of these fossils is often filled in or replaced entirely by pyrite or opal. Ammonites can still be found in large numbers along the beaches and cliffs of northeast England.

In ancient Egypt, and probably in many other old cultures, the ammonite was seen as a symbol of any deity who was connected with the ram and its curved horns. Pliny wrote that these fossils were called "*Hammonis Cornu*" and were considered sacred stones in Ethiopia. The people of that region wore the ammonite primarily to gain prophetic dreams, but also said it granted deep meditations.

During the Dark Ages in Britain, many pagan amulets and talismans were taken over by Christianity and given a Christian symbolism, simply because the people would not stop using them. One of these was the ammonite. In 656 C.E., at the Whitby Abbey in England, supposedly there lived a sainted nun whose name was Hilda. At that time the surrounding moors and the River Esk were said to be infested with poisonous snakes. St. Hilda supposedly prayed for intercession for the people, and the snakes were said to coil up, roll over the cliffs, and turn instantly into stone, thus producing ammonites. Today, these fossils are still known as St. Hilda's stones in that part of England and believed to grant miracles.

Gullible purchasers are often led to buy what they think are "snakestones," or the remains of ancient snakes, but which are actually only ammonites with a carved snake's head at one end.

Known as odontolite ("tooth stone"), bone turquoise is actually fossil teeth or bones that have been colored by the action of phosphate of iron and vivianite.

Fossils are generally associated with all five elements: Earth, Air, Fire, Water, and Spirit.

To dream of fossils can mean a static condition in life that keeps you from succeeding in your goals. If you are scattered and have not planned out goals, it can also symbolize a need to stabilize and structure your life.

▶ **HEALING ENERGIES:** Unknown.

▶ **MAGICAL POWERS:** All fossils can help with past life regression and general protection.

Ammonite: used in finding your way down the spiritual spiral path to the center where the Goddess and God await; also very useful in past-life meditations.

Bone Turquoise: useful in spells to bring something concrete into manifestation.

Copralite: aids in feeling a kinship with all other life forms.

Sand Dollar: helpful in rituals and spellworking where you want to call upon all of the elements; will add elemental powers to any spell or candle burning.

Sponge: aids in connecting with the element of Water and the entities associated with water; helpful when working to get the emotions under control.

Tigillite: heals, calms, and centers fears after experiences where your survival was in question or you were terrified.

Turitella: helps in combining the old and the new; aids in adjusting to changes in life; helps blend in new family members. Helps to neutralize fears.

MAGICAL USES

All fossils are useful to add power to spells and rituals, especially if you want all the energy of the five elements to be present. Placed on altars as focal points, around candles during burnings, hung in the house or car, or held during meditations, fossils can create a bridge to other worlds and other planes of power and existence.

Tigillite and ammonite are excellent for cross-time astral travels and/or meditations. By concentrating on the fossil's form, you can visualize yourself moving or falling along their patterns and coming out into another place.

Sand dollars, fossilized or modern, represent the five elements on any altar. The five-point star shown in their design has long been a sacred symbol and a connection with the Goddess.

The sponge can signal to the subconscious that certain factors within your life need to be mopped up and taken away.

Galena

- ► **HARDNESS:** 2.5–3
- ► **COLOR:** Silvery blue gray.
- ► **SOURCE:** Worldwide.
- ► **FACTS:** An opaque mineral and the primary ore of lead, galena cleaves into cubes or blocks. Today, most of the silver comes from ores such as galena. There is only about 2.2 pounds of silver in a ton of galena. Another modern name for this stone is galenite. Although this stone feels heavy and has a silvery appearance, it is not a metal.
- ► **HISTORY AND FOLKLORE:** Galena has been recognized as a valuable mineral containing silver and lead since ancient Roman times. Pliny gave this stone the name galena, but Aristotle called it *itmid stone.*[22]

  Galena is associated with the sign of Capricorn by some writers.

  To dream of galena means a truth will be revealed; make certain you are not guilty of exaggerating.
- ► **HEALING ENERGIES:** Unknown.
- ► **MAGICAL POWERS:** A stone for philosophers, as it promotes seeking out and telling the truth, it grounds and centers both the physical and non-physical bodies. It can also aid in astral time travel to the past.

MAGICAL USES

If you feel spacey and cannot pinpoint the cause of this feeling, sit quietly with a piece of galena in your hand. Concentrate on sending the uneasy, flighty feelings into the stone as you slowly breathe deeply in and out several times. Do not do more than ten such breaths at one sitting, or you will get light-headed.

Garnet

- ▶ **HARDNESS:** 7–7.5 (pyrope, almandine, and rhodolite). 6.5–7.5 (spessartine, grossular, andradite, hessonite, demantoid, tsavolite, and uvarovite)
- ▶ **COLORS:** Deep red-purple, yellow, brown, green, orange, flame red, reddish orange, brownish yellow, pink to rose red hues. There is one color that a garnet will never be: blue.
- ▶ **SOURCES:** (Pyrope) Arizona, South Africa, Argentina, Australia, Brazil, Myanmar, Scotland, and Switzerland. (Spessartine) Tanzania, Germany, and Italy. (Almandine) worldwide. (Uvarovite) the Ural Mountains in Russia, Finland, Turkey, Italy, and California. (Hessonite) Sri Lanka, Madagascar, Brazil, Canada, Siberia, Maine, California, New Hampshire. (Grossular) Mexico, South Africa, Canada, Sri Lanka, Pakistan, Russia, Tanzania, and the U.S.
- ▶ **FACTS:** There are several types of garnet that are considered to be of gem quality: pyrope, almandine, spessartine, grossular, andradite, rhodolite, hessonite, demantoid, tsavolite, and uvarovite. The name garnet comes from either the Latin word *granatus* ("grain-like") or *granatici* ("pomegranate"). Precious garnet is translucent, while common garnet is not.

  The garnet can range in hue from colorless to red; violet to orange; yellow to green; and brown to black, although most sold in jewelry are some shade of red.

  When miners found garnets in South Africa while digging for diamonds, they named them Cape Rubies.

  Much of the antique jewelry of the last half of the nineteenth century is set with beautiful, fiery red pyrope garnets from the ancient mines of Bohemia. This stone, which can be blood red, brick red, or dark red, seldom has inclusions and can be perfectly transparent. The name pyrope comes from the Greek word *pyropos* ("fiery"). Jewelry set with pyrope garnets has been made in Bohemia for over 500 years. In the royal jewels of Saxony is a pyrope garnet that weighs 468 1/2 carats; the Green Vaults at Dresden hold one as big as a pigeon's egg. The pyrope garnet is also called the Colorado ruby. Pyrope is found in South Africa, Zimbabwe, Tanzania, the U.S., Mexico, Brazil, Argentina, and Australia.

The almandine garnet is usually a dark, deep red-purple, sometimes appearing almost dark purple or black. Usually opaque or subtranslucent, the almandine may show a four-rayed star when cut *en cabochon*. This is caused by the inclusions of needle-like rutile or hornblende. In past centuries, slices of almandine garnet were used in the windows of temples and churches. Its name comes from *carbunculus alabandicus*, after the city of Alabanda in Asia Minor; this stone was traded in that region in the time of Pliny the Elder. Almandine is found in Sri Lanka, India, Burma, Brazil, the U.S., Madagascar, Tanzania, and Australia.

Named after the Spessartine district of Bavaria, Germany, spessartine garnet is usually bright orange, dark orange, or flame red. Its inclusions are feather-like. Only identification of the inclusions can differentiate spessartine from hessonite garnet or yellow topaz. Mandarin garnet is a bright orange spessartine discovered in only 1992 in Namibia, Africa.

One type of grossular garnet is called hessonite and mostly comes from Sri Lanka, Switzerland, and South Africa. Also called Cinnamon Stone or Essonite, this garnet can be from colorless, reddish orange, and brownish yellow, to black in color. The orange-brown of the hessonite is due to manganese and iron inclusions. The Greeks and Romans used hessonite for cameos and cabochons in jewelry. A few writers say the names jacinth and hyacinth belong to the hessonite garnet family.[23] However, most writers disagree and apply these names to zircons.

The ordinary green grossular garnet is sometimes called gooseberry, after its color. This massive stone, primarily mined in South Africa, which can be as large as a boulder, is commonly known as Transvaal Jade. It resembles jade in its coloring and appearance. Recently this type has been discovered in pink to rose red hues as well; this color of grossular garnet is called rosolite.

A transparent variety of green grossular, called tsavorite, began to be mined in only one place along a river in Kenya in the 1960s; this mine may be exhausted at any time. Chromium and vanadium give it its rich green color.

The andradite garnet called demantoid contains titanium and manganese, which give it an emerald green color. When faceted, demantoid has high fire and flashes of color. It can be recognized by the characteristic horsetail inclusions, which are actually fine, hair-like strands of asbestos. The best demantoid crystals have been found in the Ural Mountains in Russia. Only very small crystals of an andradite garnet, called topazolite, have been found; these range in color from pale to dark yellow; this variety of garnet is found in the Swiss and Italian alps. Another rare form of andradite is melanite, which is generally black; these crystals have been found on the island of Elba and in France and Germany.

Rhodolite is a deep pink or pinkish red garnet. Its name comes from the Greek words *rhodon* (rose) and *lithos* (stone). Not a common gemstone, it is found in the United States, Zimbabwe, Tanzania, and Sri Lanka.

Most people do not know that the foundations of the buildings on Manhattan Island in New York are driven deep into the bedrock that has a vast amount of garnet in it.

▶ **HISTORY AND FOLKLORE:** Ancient cultures for some reason always carved the deep red garnets *en cabochon*; any red stone carved in this manner was also called a carbuncle. *En cabochon* means that the stone was cut oval with a high dome on top and the bottom flat.

Bronze Age ruins in Czechoslovakia have yielded red garnet necklaces. The garnet was also used for gems and inlays in Egypt well before 3100 B.C.E., in Sumeria about 2300 B.C.E., and in Sweden between 2000–1000 B.C.E. It remained a popular gemstone of Greece and Rome as well as Russia into the second century C.E. A seventh century ship burial in East Anglia, England revealed garnet ornaments when it was excavated.

The garnet has long been known as the warrior's stone.

Soldiers from all over the world carried this gem as a talisman against death and injury, but it was also thought to bring victory, peace, and tranquility. Many Crusaders had a garnet set in signet rings, belt buckles, sword hilts, and shields. Ancient surgeons put the garnet on wounds to stop bleeding. This belief is still held today by soldiers and participants in violent sports in such areas as the Middle East and Asia.

In India and Persia, garnet was worn as an amulet against poison, the plague, and lightning. It was also believed to warn of approaching danger by changing color.

In Italy, the garnet is called *pietra della vedovanze* ("stone of widowhood") because widows traditionally wear it in jewelry.

Although garnet was believed to protect against deadly wounds, it was also thought to inflict them. This belief was so strong that during the fighting between the British and the Indian nationalists in 1892 the tribesmen often loaded their guns with ball-shaped garnets, which actually did inflict many serious or fatal wounds.

Greek children today still wear garnets to protect against drowning, obviously based on the garnet's reputation of keeping the wearer safe from harm.

As late as the 1600s, doctors were prescribing a "magistery" or tonic of red garnet to stimulate the heart, improve blood flow, and remove toxins. Although garnets were worn for the same reasons, the patient, particularly those with heart problems, had to remain calm as any excitement might cause great anger leading to severe health problems. Garnet was also used to treat melancholy; the depressed person, however, could expect to be plagued by insomnia.

When given as a gift, the garnet is said to grant loyalty and affection. However, when the stone loses its luster, the owner should beware of approaching danger and disaster. A stolen garnet is said to bring bad luck to the thief until it is returned to the rightful owner. The green garnet (demantoid) gives great success to the businessperson.

Garnets are connected with the signs of Virgo, Capricorn, and Aquarius, and is said to be ruled by Mars.

To dream of a garnet symbolizes the solution to a mystery was close at hand.

▶ **HEALING ENERGIES:** Purifies and regenerates all body systems, particularly the blood and heart. Considered one of the best general tonics for the entire bodily system, as well as helping with hemorrhage and infections.

Andradite (green): healing to veins.

▶ **MAGICAL POWERS:** It helps in balancing the root chakra, but also stimulates the pituitary gland. A stone that can connect with the kundalini energy of transformation, the garnet can regenerate and transmute; at the same time it can lift depression and help keep the thoughts on a higher level. Works well with rose quartz.

Can aid in bringing in business opportunities. A good protection stone, garnet can be placed under the pillow to prevent bad dreams.

Garnet can have an effect upon the pituitary and pineal glands, as well as the intuitive centers of the mind. It can be used to access information about past lives.

Almandine (red with violet tint): increases productivity; helps to stay focused and get things done. If held to the third eye, this stone can access past-life information.

Pyrope (red with brown tint): balances productivity and happiness.

Rhodolite (rose red or pale pink violet): enhances productivity and prosperity in the career.

Spessartite (orange-brown, orange, yellow-orange): focuses on productivity in the home; excellent for anyone whose career is the home; strengthens happiness and contentment.

Star garnet: high-powered productivity for long periods of time.

Tsavorite (green and rare): helps in taking control of one's life, regardless of the opinions of others. Connected with Mercury, tsavorite also helps with communications in any form, including writing. Helps in overcoming shyness and lack of confidence.

Uvarovite: This garnet was named after a professor of the late Russian Imperial Academy at what was once called Petrograd. Stimulates the imagination; improves verbal skills and charisma. Very good for anyone in the "storytelling" field.

MAGICAL USES

Wear or carry garnets whenever you feel you are or will be in a combative, very competitive situation. If you are suffering from malicious gossip and lies, wearing a garnet will send the negative vibrations right back to those perpetrating them. Whenever you feel or hear negative remarks, mentally place the garnet between you and the trouble-makers; the rebound will probably go unnoticed until they suffer the results.

Wear uvarovite if you are in the field of writing, whether it be factual, fiction, or television and movie scripts. It draws inspiration and helps give you access to new ideas.

Geodes

▶ **HARDNESS:** 7

▶ **COLORS:** Exterior of a tan or brown; interior contains crystals of quartz, amethyst, or similar gemstones.

▶ **SOURCE:** Worldwide.

▶ **FACTS:** Geodes come in two kinds—hollow nodules with crystal centers or a solid stone with a center of mineral deposits, usually of agate—and are unique and individual. Found most frequently in rocks consisting largely of silicon and calcium minerals, the most recognized type of geode is a rock cavity lined with crystals. These crystals can be clear quartz or amethyst.

When a closed geode is broken open, it often contains water from the time of its forming. Geodes are also formed in existing cavities, shells, or fossils. Elongated hollow geodes are called "logs"; these are very expensive.

Thunder eggs, or solid agate nodules with a star-like interior, are found frequently in Oregon. The solid minerals filling thunder eggs can be agate, jasper, sardonyx, or even other minerals.

Brazil yields many of the best geodes. At one time, miners found an amethyst geode that was over 30 feet long and 15 feet high. This geode alone held 700 tons of what is known as "first-sized" amethysts.

▶ **HISTORY AND FOLKLORE:** Also known as thunder eggs, echites, eagle stone, and aetites. Another name for the geode is the potato stone, probably from its rough appearance before the inner beauty is revealed.

The geode is sometimes associated with Gemini.

To dream of a geode symbolizes a truth or beauty of a person or situation that will be revealed if you are patient and look closely.

▶ **HEALING ENERGIES:** Unknown.

▶ **MAGICAL POWERS:** Each geode represents a different observation of some truth. Oftentimes, this truth is recalling correctly your past lives. Geodes are extremely useful for past-life meditations.

Use to concentrate your magical power just before releasing it. Can also be used as a focus point for going across time.

If two halves of a geode are shared between friends, the energy flow between the two halves will remain linked.

MAGICAL USES

Use a geode as a focal point for past-life exploration in meditation. However, you must be very careful that you are not seeing what you want to see, but seeing only what is true.

A geode is also useful when you are dealing with tough experiences that make you wish you could hide out in a hole or cave somewhere. Hold the geode and visualize yourself shrinking and going into the cave-like stone. Feel the crystals pulling out all the hurt and frustration and loneliness. Feel the stones filling you with gentle energy and strength.

Goldstone

▶ **HARDNESS:** 6

▶ **COLORS:** A semitransparent brown color with spots of golden yellow mica. Also a blue with copper flecks.

▶ **SOURCES:** Natural stone; also one variety is manmade.

▶ **FACTS:** A member of the oligoclase family of minerals; a type of quartz.

A simulated product known as Oregon goldstone contains tiny pieces of copper sealed in glass; this is a beautiful coppery, gold color.

▶ **HISTORY AND FOLKLORE:** Pliny was familiar with goldstone under the name of *sandaresus* ("stars of gold gleaming within"). The Germans know the simulated version of this stone under the name of *Goldfluss*.

Goldstone is under the sign of Leo.

To dream of goldstone signifies that you need to look closely at a person or situation. You may be blinded by illusion and not seeing the truth, whether this is negative or positive.

▶ **HEALING ENERGIES:** Unknown.

▶ **MAGICAL POWERS:** Useful in raising one's energy frequency. Raises the energy levels.

MAGICAL USES

Carry or wear goldstone to help keep your energy levels high during very busy times. This stone will also add to the energy level of a ritual or spell if placed on the altar or in your sacred place.

Goshenite

▶ **HARDNESS:** 7.5

▶ **COLOR:** Colorless.

▶ **SOURCES:** Massachusetts, Canada, Brazil, and Russia.

▶ **FACTS:** A pure, colorless form of beryl, goshenite has been used to imitate diamond or emerald.

▶ **HISTORY AND FOLKLORE:** Goshenite got its name from Goshen, Massachusetts, where it was first found and recognized as a new stone.

At one time goshenite was used for spectacle lenses. The German word *brille* ("spectacles") may have been derived from the word beryl.

This stone is connected with Pisces.

To dream of goshenite symbolizes a need to be less stubborn.

▶ **HEALING ENERGIES:** Unknown.'

▶ **MAGICAL POWERS:** Lessens stubbornness and balances those with little or no emotional empathy for others. Good for those who get into an intellectual rut and cannot change their opinions.

MAGICAL USES

If you find yourself in a spiritual rut, as well as a mental and physical one, you need to do something to break through the blockages you have erected within your subconscious mind. This must take place on a twofold level.

First, you have to become aware of every time you say or do something out of habit, a reaction that is based primarily on stubbornness and resistance to change. Each night go over your day and write down every incident that has this underlying resistance to it. Carefully think over why you reacted as you did. Was it because of a past event? Is it connected with impressions and learned responses from childhood? Is there another legitimate way of understanding the event, other than the view you held?

The second part of this self-treatment is to do twice-weekly meditations. Gaze at a piece of goshenite just before going into meditation. See yourself going through the stone and out the other side, into a secure place where your guides can communicate with you. As you go through the stone, feel your resistance to change being pulled away. The other side of the stone will reveal only truth, so your subconscious illusions and excuses will not be valid there. You can call up any event in your life, see it from the outside, and begin to understand both sides of any experience.

Hawk's-Eye

▶ **HARDNESS:** 7

▶ **COLORS:** Blue gray or bluish.

▶ **SOURCE:** Primarily from South Africa.

▶ **FACTS:** Hawk's-eye is a quartz with fibrous inclusions. When cut *en cabochon*, these inclusions produce chatoyancy, or an eye-like effect. Less common than quartz cat's-eye, tiger's-eye, or bull's-eye, this stone is more expensive than its relatives are. Although there are cheap-looking glass imitations of the quartz eye stones on the market, these stones have never been successfully synthetically produced.

▶ **HISTORY AND FOLKLORE:** None known.

Hawk's-eye is associated with the element of Air and the sign of Scorpio.

To dream of this stone means you need to set goals for the future.

▶ **HEALING ENERGIES:** Unknown.

▶ **MAGICAL POWERS:** Helps you to get back on the right path; use it for regaining control of your life and activities.

Can be used for divination.

MAGICAL USES

If you feel blocked or frustrated with the way your life and/or goals are turning out, and want to look into the future to see what changes could be made, use the hawk's-eye stone. Hold the stone to your third eye in the center of your forehead. Close your eyes and relax, looking inwardly toward the hawk's-eye and your third eye. Mentally affirm what you need to see in order to make changes. At first you may only see flashes of colors or light, but soon these will form into pictures. You may well get other clues to help you in dreams.

Heliodor

▶ **HARDNESS:** 7.5–8

▶ **COLORS:** Yellow, golden yellow.

▶ **SOURCES:** The Ural Mountains in Russia, Brazil, Madagascar, the Ukraine, Namibia, and the U.S.

▶ **FACTS:** The golden variety of beryl, heliodor has always been linked to the Sun and it takes its name from that celestial body. Although gem-quality specimens are occasionally found, most heliodor has inclusions of fine, slender tubes. It is often found along with aquamarine.

▶ **HISTORY AND FOLKLORE:** None known.

Heliodor is associated with the Sun and the sign of Leo.

To dream of heliodor foretells success and recognition.

▶ **HEALING ENERGIES:** Clears the body of toxins.

▶ **MAGICAL POWERS:** A comforting stone, it helps one to empathize with others and feel comfortable doing it. Also a high energy stone, heliodor resonates with the pituitary gland and aids in spiritual and psychic development.

MAGICAL USES

This is a good stone to wear if you are having difficulty understanding the problems of a close friend or relative. By holding the stone in your power hand while with this person, you can feel her/his emotional needs and better understand what is upsetting or troubling her/him. To avoid cording, or the attaching of energy lines from this person to your aura, also wear a piece of red jasper. Later ground yourself with clear quartz or one of the stones associated with the element of Earth.

Keep a heliodor on your altar or with your meditation equipment to aid in developing your psychic powers and spiritual communications.

Hematite

▶ **HARDNESS:** 6.5

▶ **COLORS:** An opaque, massive black or dark iron-gray stone with a metallic luster; shows a blood red color when sliced thin or powdered.

▶ **SOURCES:** Canada, Brazil, Venezuela, England, Switzerland, Germany, Spain, the U.S., and Elba.

▶ **FACTS:** The word hematite probably comes from the Greek words *haima, aima, haimatites,* or *ema,* meaning blood or blood-like, because of its red-colored dust. Sometimes called bloodstone, it was associated with Mars, the god of war. Hematite is the same stone as specularite.

An imitation substance, hematine, which closely resembles hematite, is made of stainless steel, chromium, and nickel sulfides. However, hematine is magnetic, while natural hematite is not.[24]

On occasion, iridescent hematite crystals, called iron roses, are found, primarily in sites in Switzerland and Brazil. These short, black crystals with their rainbow iridescence are arranged almost like the petals of a flower.

Most marcasite jewelry today is actually faceted hematite. Actual marcasite tends to erode and dissolve from exposure to the air.

▶ **HISTORY AND FOLKLORE:** During the early Iron Age, hematite was considered to be almost as valuable as gold. One of the oldest surviving Babylonian gem treatises, written by Azchalias for Mithridates the Great (king of Pontus 63 B.C.E.), mentions the virtues and uses of hematite. It was worn to gain favorable hearings during judgments and lawsuits, to win positive petitions before all those in authority, and to protect warriors. Hematite was used in Babylon, Assyria, and other ancient civilizations as far back as 2000 B.C.E. The Egyptians used hematite pillows for the heads of the dead to rest upon. Pieces of engraved hematite have also been found in tombs, as well as ancient Babylonian mines.

In the ancient Roman culture, both hematite and iron were sacred to the god Mars. Roman soldiers and gladiators wore this stone for protection against battle wounds. The Spartans, who put childbirth on par with war, used hematite for birth and delivery.

When Hitler came to power in Germany, the Nazi party used hematite as their symbol, representing "blood and iron."[25]

When scraped, this stone produces a blood red powder, which ancient physicians used to stop bleeding of all kinds, whether external or internal. It was also given for urinary problems. In the Sudan in Africa, hematite was worn to prevent headaches and sunstroke.

This stone is sometimes called black diamond, although it is not a diamond, nor does it have the diamond's hardness and other characteristics. Today, hematite is frequently faceted and sold as marcasite.

Hematite is associated with the signs of Aries and Aquarius.

To dream of this stone symbolizes a need for grounding and balance in your life.

▶ **HEALING ENERGIES:** Increases resistance to stress as well as strengthening the blood and spleen. Use for bloodshot eyes, to relieve headaches, and prevent heat stroke in the summer. Used to draw illnesses out of the body by placing on the diseased part.

▶ **MAGICAL POWERS:** Energizes the etheric body and helps to give optimism, will, and courage. Will help in grounding, but only for certain people. Helps in reevaluation of personal issues and life patterns. Helps to obtain a favorable outcome of lawsuits and judgments.

Because it can repel and dissolve negativity, hematite is sometimes called the anti-stress stone. Reduces stress by breaking up and destroying negativity. Strengthens all the bodies. Good for focusing on past lives.

MAGICAL USES

Carry hematite and stroke it as you would a worry stone to release stress and dissolve negativity. If you have a modern piece of jewelry that has "marcasite" in it, you are really wearing hematite. Combined with other stones in this manner, the small pieces of faceted hematite do an excellent job of breaking up incoming negative vibrations and reflecting them away from you, while the larger and different stone will work according to its special powers. If you should happen to acquire a ring of garnet and marcasite (hematite), for example, you have two protective stones working together.

Because hematite has a shiny, reflective surface, this stone can also be used as a scrying device. Let soft light, such as from a candle, shine on the stone while gazing at its surface. The pictures may be shown within the stone or may appear in your mind.

Hiddenite

▶ **HARDNESS:** 6–7
▶ **COLORS:** Shades and intensities of emerald green; sometimes yellow.

▶ **SOURCE:** Brazil, Madagascar, Myanmar, the U.S., Canada, Russia, Mexico, and Sweden.

▶ **FACTS:** Hiddenite was named after W. E. Hidden, who first discovered it in North Carolina in 1881. A member of the mineral group spodumene, hiddenite is fragile because of its perfect cleavage. Because of this tendency to shatter, hiddenite is most often sold without being cut or faceted. Sometimes called Lithia Emerald, this stone is rarer than the lilac-pink kunzite, which is also a member of this group. This is because of the chromium that is needed to give it the green color.

▶ **HISTORY AND FOLKLORE:** None known.

Hiddenite is sometimes connected with Pluto.

To dream of hiddenite signifies a fragile situation that could shatter if the right actions and words are not carefully used.

▶ **HEALING ENERGIES:** Unknown.

▶ **MAGICAL POWERS:** Excellent for spiritual awareness and connecting with the universe. Balances the higher centers and bodies.

MAGICAL USES

Hold a piece of hiddenite to the throat chakra, the third eye, and the crown chakra for about two minutes in each place. This will help to clear these upper light centers and open them to higher spiritual awareness. Do not keep the stone on these chakras for longer than two minutes, as it may make you very nervous and restless.

Holey Stones

▶ **SOURCE:** Worldwide.

▶ **FACTS:** A holey stone can be any type of stone with a naturally occurring hole worn through it by the action of Nature. Called holed stones, holey stones, holy stones, or Odhinn Stones.

▶ **HISTORY AND FOLKLORE:** Stones that have natural holes have always been considered magical and sacred, with special healing properties. Many of the larger European holey stones are still used by people as a cure for certain illnesses, such as rheumatism, arthritis, and childhood diseases. The sick person had to crawl through the hole in order to lose the disease.

Holey stones are connected with the element of Earth.

To dream of a holey stone symbolizes an approaching spiritual experience that will leave you and your life changed.

▶ **HEALING ENERGIES:** Draws out illnesses if run through the aura.

▶ **MAGICAL POWERS:** Carry a small holey stone for luck and to ward off evil magic. Hanging one over the bed will prevent nightmares. Placing these stones around the house or hanging one over the door will protect the house and its occupants from harm.

Look through a holey stone by moonlight to see visions, ghosts, or non-physical beings.

MAGICAL USES

Hang a holey stone over the head of the bed by a red ribbon to prevent nightmares. Used in this manner, the stone acts much the same as a dream catcher. Just remember to periodically cleanse the stone, as it will eventually get full.

Look through the hole in the stone while standing in moonlight. A little practice will reveal the flitting forms of the Fairy Folk and Nature spirits, especially if you are outside during the time of a Full Moon.

If you are under magical attack, hang a holey stone by a black ribbon over the front door, or whichever door is regularly used in the home. This snags negative vibrations as soon as they enter.

Hold a holey stone to the third eye at the beginning of meditation to make contact with your teachers and guides.

Iolite

▶ **HARDNESS:** 7–7.5
▶ **COLOR:** violet blue.
▶ **SOURCES:** Sri Lanka, Myanmar, Madagascar, India, Namibia, Tanzania, Germany, Norway, and Finland.
▶ **FACTS:** Also known as cordierite and Indialite, iolite is sometimes

called water sapphire. It is dichroic, appearing colorless from one direction, colored from another.

▶ **HISTORY AND FOLKLORE:** The name iolite comes from the Greek words *ion* ("violet") and *lithos* ("stone").

Iolite is often associated with Aquarius.

To dream of iolite means an unexpected solution to a difficult problem.

▶ **HEALING ENERGIES:** Unknown.

▶ **MAGICAL POWERS:** Good for submissive people as this stone strengthens self-confidence and taking charge of life. Projects anti-martyr and anti-victim vibrations. Helps one feel comfortable in taking a leadership role. Attracts friends and friendly help.

Aids in moving the thoughts into a higher realm.

MAGICAL USES

If you wish to find new friends, iolite can be helpful. Write out the basic qualities you want in a friend. Fold this paper around a piece of iolite and tie it with a blue thread. Place the wrapped stone on your altar with pieces of crystal to the four directions around it. Set a small vase of flowers behind this stone formation. Each day burn a blue candle for fifteen minutes, using the same candle until it is completely gone. Then unwrap the iolite and burn the paper. Carry the stone with you until you have attracted all the friends you want. Remember that no ritual will do all the work. You still have to be friendly and get out to appropriate gatherings and places where you can meet people.

Ivory

▶ **HARDNESS:** 2.5–2.75

▶ **COLOR:** Ivory, cream.

▶ **SOURCE:** Taken from both land and marine animals, such as elephant, hippopotamus, boar, warthog, walrus, and sea lion.

▶ **FACTS:** If you wish to own ivory, please see that you buy it from legitimate sources, such as the Eskimo or certain African nations, who have the right to harvest it. Otherwise, purchase old, antique pieces.

Fossil ivory is also available and comes from such creatures as the dinosaur, mastodon, and mammoth. Excavators in France found one piece of mammoth ivory that has been estimated to be over 30,000 years old.

► **HISTORY AND FOLKLORE:** Ivory has been used and carved for thousands of years. It was quite popular for jewelry and ornaments. Ivory substitutes, such as bone, vegetable ivory, and horn, are now used instead. Forms of vegetable ivory are the seed of the Doum palm from Africa and those of the Corozo nuts of South America.

Ivory is often associated with Uranus and the sign of Libra.

To dream of ivory symbolizes your need to break free of a person, job, or situation that is demoralizing or demeaning in some way.

► **HEALING ENERGIES:** Balances and heals all chakras.

► **MAGICAL POWERS:** Stabilizes and balances the energy levels by purifying the aura. Especially helpful to those who have a low self-worth by calming and lifting the mood.

MAGICAL USES

Although some writers absolutely will not consider using any kind of ivory at all, I believe in the use of legitimately sold ivory. The best use I have found for ivory is to contact animal helpers from the spirit realms. By wearing or holding a piece of ivory while on a shamanic journey you can contact and communicate with your animal allies much easier. This is of great help if you have had difficulty making previous contacts.

When you first acquire a piece of ivory, it will definitely need to be cleaned of vibrations. Do not use salt; instead hold the ivory under cool running water, dry carefully, and then hold it in the smoke of frankincense incense.

Jade

▶ **HARDNESS:** 6.5–7 (Jadeite). 5–6.5 (Nephrite)

▶ **COLORS:** Apple green, white, pink, yellow, mauve, black, gray, brown.

▶ **SOURCE:** (Jadeite) Myanmar, Guatemala, Japan, and California. (Nephrite) Myanmar, Siberia, Russia, China, North and South Islands of New Zealand, Turkestan, Central Asia, Australia, Canada, Mexico, Brazil, Taiwan, Zimbabwe, Italy, Poland, Germany, Switzerland, the U.S., and Tibet.

▶ **FACTS:** Jade was thought to be just one type of stone until the 1800s when it was discovered that there were two kinds of jade: jadeite and nephrite. Very similar in appearance, both jades are hard and fine. However, jadeite is the hardest and more finely grained. Its colors range from the commonly known apple green through white, pink, yellow, mauve, and black. The apple green jade is extremely rare, and at one time all of this color and the color yellow were confiscated by the Chinese royal family. Thus it became known as Imperial Jade. Imperial Jade is quite translucent.

Nephrite is included in the hornblende group, although, like jadeite, its crystal system is monoclinic. Its colors range from green, gray, or white, to brown and yellow.

Nephrite is often called New Zealand Jade and is more widespread than jadeite. The New Zealand Maoris called it *punamu* ("green stone"); it was so rare that they used a wizard (*tohunga*) to locate it. They carve their favorite talisman, the Tiki, from jade.

The Chinese knew nephrite, which came from Turkestan, as *Yu*, a term they applied to all precious gemstones. One rich emerald green variety was called *feits 'ui* (Imperial Jade). The excavation of ancient Chinese tombs has revealed many jade pieces called *hanyu* (mouth-jade); these were placed in the mouths of the dead for protection.

Jade carvers in China had to depend upon the importation of raw jade from Burma, Turkestan, or the Kuen-Lun Mountains for carving. These were the only known jade mines, until nephrite was discovered in the mid-nineteenth century in rivers near the end of Siberia's Lake Baikal.

The word jade was not used until the conquest of South America by the Spanish. There, they found the Aztecs, Toltecs, and Omecs using the green nephrite as a cure for kidney diseases. So the Spaniards called the stone *piedra de ijada*, which means "hip stone."

► **HISTORY AND FOLKLORE:** In the Assyrio-Babylonian legend of the descent of the goddess Ishtar to the Underworld, she had to leave one article of clothing or jewelry at each of seven gates. At the fifth gate, the legend says Ishtar removed her girdle of jade, the stone that helped with childbirth. Jade was the stone worn and used by many ancient midwives. It may have been this connection of jade with the abdomen that led the second century physician Galen to wear a nephrite necklace for stomach problems.

The ancient Egyptians knew of and used jade in many religious contexts. They believed that its mystical qualities connected it to Maat, Goddess of Truth. When given as a gift, they said it brought very good fortune.

To the Chinese, jade was known as the congealed semen of the Celestial Dragon.[26] In records as early as 500 C.E., Chinese doctors were prescribing finely powdered jade taken in fruit juice for heartburn, asthma, diabetes, anxieties, strengthening the voice, and making the hair glossy. There are also surviving records telling how to make a divine liquor to stop decomposition of the body after death. Jade was boiled in a copper pot together with rice and dew water, then given to the dying.

Centuries later in Europe, physicians were using pieces of jade tied to certain areas of the body for a number of other illnesses. Purple nephrite with bands of yellow was said to help the spleen, while jade with yellow stains and deep purple splotches treated the liver. Green nephrite was tied to the feet and legs for swelling and to the lower back for kidney stones. Even in the seventeenth century, jade was being tied to the hip or hung about the neck to cause the expulsion of kidney stones and cure stomach pains.

In China and other areas of the Far East, jade bangles and amulets are widely worn to gain physical strength and throw off illnesses. Jade carved in the shape of a padlock is said to protect children from sickness, while jade butterflies are exchanged between engaged couples to ensure happiness. One Chinese royal court had a set of chimes made of jade slabs. These chimes were struck to notify those in court of events taking place and as part of religious ceremonies held there. Green jade is said to bring rain and drive away evil spirits. The Chinese carved jade into the shapes of bats and storks as a symbol of long life.

The Greeks and Romans wore jade to avoid stomach problems and kidney stones. Jade is still very popular with racing enthusiasts as a stone that draws success.

Jade is associated with the signs of Aries, Gemini, and Libra.

To dream of jade can mean a health problem that needs attention. It can also mean the approach of an experience that will forcibly move you out of a rut or decision that you can no longer avoided making.

▶ **HEALING ENERGIES:** Strengthens the heart, kidneys, and immune system by cleansing the blood. Healing powers correspond to the color of the jade. Helps with eye and female problems. The most respected stone in the Orient, jade has powerful calming vibrations. *Yellow:* helps with poor digestion.

▶ **MAGICAL POWERS:** Increases fertility in all areas. Powerful for balancing the emotions as it dispels negativity and attracts courage, justice, and wisdom. Its subtle vibrations work over a long period of time, rather than quickly. Helps to remember dreams and solve problems through your dreams. Jade is an excellent stone for business people and musicians.

Black: wear when feeling under attack and your survival is in question; opens and balances the first three chakras; also gives strength. Black jade mixed with bright green is known as chloromelanite; this is very balancing to women.

Blue: helps to neutralize karmic influences and the emotional issues tied to them; good for relaxing and meditation.

Brown or gray: calms and drains off excessive energy; temporarily lessens the impact of karmic events. Helps with adjusting to new surroundings; settles negative home matters.

Green: creates calm, peace, and harmony; counteracts depression; banishes evil spirits. Sometimes called the Dream Stone, as it produces vivid and accurate dreams.

Lavender: helps with creativity and ideas. Brings psychic understanding of dreams. Aids in recovering from a negative love.

Orange or pink: creates healthy skepticism.

Red: helps in handling angry feelings; releases tension.

White: extremely calming and grounding. Aids in making decisions.

Yellow: helps one to understand the opposite sex. Gold or red jade will attract master teachings through dreams.

MAGICAL USES

If you are experiencing a bad time dealing with emotional karmic issues, use a piece of blue, brown, or gray jade as a touchstone or worry stone. Rub the jade whenever you begin to get upset and find your emotions getting out of control. This will drain off the excess emotions and energy you feel. To be finished with the problem, however, you must detach from your emotions and look at the situation realistically. Determine what your part has been in the past life and still is now. See the lesson you should learn and acknowledge it. Only in this way can you begin to break free.

If you want to have vivid dreams, sleep with green jade under your pillow. However, if you want to be able to understand the meaning of psychic dreams, put a piece of lavender jade under the pillow with the green. Gold jade will help to attract an important spiritual teacher during your dream time.

To cover most of life's difficulties and help you in dealing with them, purchase a jade bracelet of several colors.

Jasper

▶ **HARDNESS:** 7

▶ **COLORS:** Shades of brown, grayish blue, red, yellow, green, and mixtures of these.

▶ **SOURCES:** Found in the U.S., Russia, India, Venezuela, France, Germany, and other places around the world.

▶ **FACTS:** A variety of chalcedony that is massive and fine-grained. Ribbon jasper is striped, while orbicular jasper is red with white or gray eye-shaped patterns. Hornstone is a gray variety of jasper. If jasper contains hematite, it is called jaspillite. Brown jasper with yellow flecks is vabanite. "Egyptian pebbles" is the name for yellow-brown jasper nodules, while eye-spot jasper can be labeled as kinradite. When green jasper is flecked with red spots, it is known as bloodstone, or heliotrope. Plain green jasper can be difficult to distinguish from jade.

▶ **HISTORY AND FOLKLORE:** The name jasper is said to come from the Hebrew word *yashpheh,* the Greek *iaspis,* or the Arabic *yash.* The Lydian Stone (*lapis lydius*) of ancient writers was black, flinty jasper, also called a touchstone. Pliny himself listed ten varieties of jasper, while the writer Marbodus, in his book *Lapidarium,* detailed seventeen.

All forms of jasper were held in high regard by the ancients. The oldest ornaments made of jasper, found in France, date back to the Paleolithic era (20,000–16,000 B.C.E.). Babylonian seals, dating back to 1000 B.C.E., also have been found in old ruins. The remains of the Harappa culture of India yielded magnificent jewelry containing this stone. Engraved rings of jasper have been recovered from the ruins of Pompeii, Herculaneum, and other ancient cities.

The anodyne necklace, which was so valued in England at one time, was really a necklace of jasper, worn to treat stomach troubles. Green jasper was said to grant good luck when buying or selling something.

In ancient times, jasper was believed to bring rain and cure snakebite. From the descriptions given by ancient writers, one can identify the Pantheros stone as the mottle brown Egyptian jasper. The Egyptians used it to protect against all enemies, wild animals, and fear. Jasper worn in the navel has been considered a cure for stomachaches for thousands of years. The Persians powdered this stone, along with turquoise, for the treatment of gall bladder, liver, and kidney diseases.

This stone is connected with the sign of Leo by some writers.

Dreaming about jasper means your love will be returned by a trustworthy person.

▶ **HEALING ENERGIES:** A powerful healer, it strengthens the liver and gallbladder and is soothing to the stomach and nerves.

Pink or yellow: good for hormone balancing.

Red: helps to control excessive bleeding.

Variegated: one of the strongest healing stones for the entire body. Jasper placed on the abdomen is also said to make childbirth easier.

▶ **MAGICAL POWERS:** Works on the chakras according to the color of the stone. Drives away evil spirits, hallucinations, and nightmares. A stone that works primarily on the physical body, jasper can protect and ground. Helps you to keep your feet on the ground and not get caught in extremes of emotions.

Jasper's vibrations are very subtle and are used for long-term changes, rather than quick ones. It works well with opal, supplementing and balancing the opal's powers.

Black: wear it when you want people to leave you alone; good for personal sacred and ritual places.

Brick red: sometimes called the "mother of all stones" and the first transformer because of its magical properties. Balances all chakras; stabilizes the energy levels. Protects the wearer from negativity by absorbing vibrations.

Bright green: helps to keep one cool and calculating when needed.

Brown: keeps away undesired psychic attachments or cordings. Grounds and stabilizes.

Gray: helps to regain and/or use your personal power; balances and protects the third chakra.

Green: creates balance out of extremes; removes energy blocks; clears and balances all chakras; a healer.

Picture: aids in recalling past experiences or lives that have a bearing on present problems.

Purplish red (imperial): very good for those who are unfocused.

True red: creates a sense of power and helps one to avoid being a victim. Good for defensive magic when negative energies must be returned.

MAGICAL USES

The brick red jasper is an excellent magical energizer. It adds volumes of power, whether it is a simple, "Goddess, please hold that parking place!" or a complicated and concentrated ritual. Like the true red color, the brick red is also a top-notch shield when under negative magical attack. Rather than one big burst of force, jasper builds up and maintains a steady energy for longer periods of time than most other stones.

Picture jasper works best if it has been shaped and polished, rather than left in the natural state. This brings out the "picture" design of the stone. To gain information about past lives, concentrate on ethereal design of the stone, letting your mind relax and send up whatever messages it will. Although not as detailed as past life meditations, using picture jasper will give you clues to your past-lives, clues that you can later investigate further.

Jet

- ▶ **HARDNESS:** 2.5
- ▶ **COLORS:** Waxy black or dark brown.
- ▶ **SOURCES:** England, Spain, France, Germany, Poland, India, Turkey, Russia, China, and the U.S.
- ▶ **FACTS:** Jet is actually wood that has been buried for millions of years and compressed into a type of fossil. It has a waxy dark luster and sometimes contains small pyrite inclusions that give it a metallic color. On occasion, jet will be found with embedded fossils, such as the ammonite and bivalve. If rubbed with a cloth, jet will become charged with static electricity and attract small pieces of paper, much the same as amber does. A sixteenth century writer even called it Black Amber. It takes a high polish and once was quite fashionable in jewelry, especially when Queen Victoria began to wear jet as mourning jewelry in 1861.

Excavations in the Paleolithic caves near Thayngen, Switzerland, have unearthed many pieces of jet. Pierced jet beads were also found in Belgian caves of the same era. Both jet and amber were thought to have talismanic virtues very early in human cultures.

Jet has been found in large quantities in the Whitby area of Britain since the Bronze Age. First the Romans, then the Vikings, mined British jet extensively for its magical and medicinal qualities.

Beginning in the 1600s and extending well into Victorian times, jet was first principally used to make rosaries and crucifixes, then carved into bracelets, earrings, hair ornaments, cameo rings, brooches, and other jewelry. Whitby in Yorkshire, England, was a historic source of jet, which was mined well into the nineteenth century when jet was popular as mourning jewelry.

Like amber, jet is lightweight and feels like plastic. Because of this appearance, jet should be purchased from a reputable dealer to avoid getting fake jet. Cannel coal has been made into carved items and sold as jet, but this substance can easily be distinguished from jet by its slight brownish tinge. Other substitutes used to imitate jet are anthracite, hard rubber, obsidian, black-dyed chalcedony, plastic, and a black glass called "Paris jet."

▶ **HISTORY AND FOLKLORE:** Archaeological evidence shows that jet has been mined and used since c. 1400 B.C.E. Many pieces of worked jet have been recovered from prehistoric burial mounds. When the Romans occupied Britain, jet was mined, worked, and sent to Rome.

The use of jet in magic was handed down for centuries from one magician to another. In the writings of Pliny and Bede, we find references to the burning of jet to drive off snakes or, when used in spells of acquisition, to gain desires. Pliny also said that the fumes could confirm or deny a state of virginity, although he does not say how this was done. The Greeks dedicated jet to the goddess Cybele and wore this stone when seeking a favor from the goddess.

In the Mediterranean area, jet was known as gaggitis and galaktite, because it was found at Gagge or Gagas in Lydia, according to Pliny. The Germans know this stone as *Gaget*.[27]

In Italy, as in the British Isles, jet was burned to drive away snakes and demons, protect from thunderstorms and demonical possession, and ensure the safety of an absent family member. The Italians wore jet beetles to protect against the evil eye, just as the people of India and Egypt wore little jet disks for similar protection.

Ancient physicians powdered jet and added it to wine or water as a cure for toothache and scrofula.

An ancient tradition says that when one wears jet and amber jewelry, these ornaments become part of the body and soul of the wearer. Many Wiccan priestesses wear necklaces of amber and jet.

Some writers associate jet with Saturn and the sign of Capricorn.

To dream of jet means an upcoming period where events will be depressing.

▶ **HEALING ENERGIES:** Eases headache pain behind the eyes.

▶ **MAGICAL POWERS:** Helps the wearer to be alert to all things and quickly come up with constructive solutions.

Associated with chthonic or Underworld powers, jet is said to control all demons and thus prevent demonic possession. Jet draws out negative energy from the aura, fights depression, and can initiate psychic experiences. Uncovers past negative energies a person still carries in her/his subconscious mind. Helps in understanding and working with life and karmic cycles.

A highly regarded magical stone, jet is associated with Saturn. Use it to gain victory and control over an enemy, but only in a positive manner or you will get a painful backlash of energy.

Wear amber and jet together when seeking the Goddess and asking for Her aid.

MAGICAL USES

Some people have a dislike for or uneasy feeling when working with black and/or Saturn stones. I like the Saturn stones and have no problem working with them; I also like and respect the Crone aspect of the Goddess, an aspect also linked with black stones. I have always liked these stones, so my feelings have nothing to do with my age. It has been my observation that if you have a problem using black or Saturn stones, you need to work on karmic issues you have avoided.

Jet adds a wonderful, deep spiritual dimension when used or worn during rituals. It can induce dreams of important karmic influences at work in your life. With its strong Crone connections, jet can help you come to terms with aging and the elder people in your life. If you have suffered a loss through death, it can also comfort and ease the pain.

Kunzite

► **HARDNESS:** 6–7
► **COLOR:** Lilac-pink.
► **SOURCES:** Brazil, Madagascar, Myanmar, the U.S., Canada, Russia, Mexico, and Sweden.
► **FACTS:** A member of the mineral group spodumene, kunzite was discovered in the early twentieth century and is named after the gemologist George F. Kunz. Kunzite and hiddenite were not recognized as separate gemstones until 1879. Kunzite, colored by manganese, is fragile with perfect cleavage. It is also dichroic, that is, a deeper color when viewed from one direction than from another. The lilac-pink color of some stones may fade with time.[28] It is, however, an expensive stone.

When yellowish or colorless, the stone is called triphane. When it is emerald green, it is given the name of hiddenite. It is a non-conductor of electricity and will fluoresce a pale orange under ultraviolet light.
► **HISTORY AND FOLKLORE:** None known.

Kunzite is associated with Venus and Taurus.

To dream of kunzite reveals a need to stop avoiding unpleasant issues and solve them.
► **HEALING ENERGIES:** Will ease tension of tight muscles. Especially good for the nerves and muscles of the shoulders and neck.
► **MAGICAL POWERS:** Creates calmness when you have to accept a situation because it is out of your control.

Kunzite is connected with the heart, or fourth chakra and promotes emotional balance. It can be used to remove emotional blockages built from past experiences. Use kunzite with rose quartz to reveal, bring up, and dissolve buried childhood experiences of deep emotional stress.

MAGICAL USES

Since this stone is fairly new, its range of magical energies is still being explored.

Kunzite can be used in love spells. However, it will promote more of a spiritual love, than one of the physical variety. Used as a worry stone, it can drain away excess restlessness and nervousness if held in your receiving hand (not the hand with which you write).

One of the best uses of kunzite is for the removal of subconscious emotional blockages from past experiences. We all carry around this buried garbage and need to clean it out before we can move on to better things. Hold during meditation to see what the problems are, or, if you are really determined, sleep with kunzite under your pillow with the same result in mind. Your dreams may be unsettling, however, until you face and take steps to do away with the emotional baggage.

Labradorite

▶ **HARDNESS:** 6–6.5

▶ **COLORS:** Most commonly silver gray or blue gray with an iridescence on the dark ground, but can be colorless, orange, yellow, or red.

▶ **SOURCES:** Labrador in Canada, Finland, Norway, and Russia.

▶ **FACTS:** Named after St. Paul Island, Labrador, where it was first identified in 1770, labradorite has a play of color (schiller) when the stone is moved in the light. The metallic play of colors, or labradorescence as it is called, reminds one of the silvery blue-green reflections on fish scales or a butterfly wing. The ground color is usually a shade of dark smoky gray, but the inclusions of rutile, ilmenite, and magnetite cause rainbow-colored reflections when the light strikes the stone.

This stone is the plagioclase feldspar and in the same family as albite. Labradorite has been found in some meteorites.

Gem-quality labradorite is known as spectrolite, while a colorless variety, darkened with needlelike inclusions, is often called black moonstone.[29] Spectrolite is a dark, opalescent blue with shimmer when the light hits it. It was discovered in Finland during World War II. Another name for this stone is falcon's-eye.

▶ **HISTORY AND FOLKLORE:** Pieces of labradorite have been discovered among the artifacts of the Red Painted People of Maine; these date back long before the year C.E. 1000.

There is no ancient history known about spectrolite.

Labradorite is associated with the signs of Sagittarius, Scorpio, and Leo, while spectrolite is connected with the Moon, Uranus, and Aquarius.

To dream of labradorite symbolizes a subconscious need to connect with your creative, spiritual side. To dream of spectrolite means the unveiling of hidden mysteries.

▶ **HEALING ENERGIES:** Unknown.

▶ **MAGICAL POWERS:** Labradorite is excellent for those who overwork or those who are facing a period of sustained work. Stimulates physical activity, the willingness to get into action.

Labradorite also lifts the consciousness and can establish a connection with the universal energies.

Spectrolite can protect and balance the entire aura. It helps cultivate patience and perseverance. Use in spellwork for manifesting results to improbable situations.

MAGICAL USES

Labradorite seems to have the strongest effect on the fifth, sixth, and seventh chakras. A stone that subtly affects the way you respond to situations, mentally and physically, this stone can be worn often without tiring results.

Spectrolite, however, has a totally different vibration. Simply wearing spectrolite in jewelry can be an intense experience. It forces open the subconscious mind and allows ideas to bubble up. It can bring in unexpected and unlikely solutions that take you by surprise; this can be pleasant or unpleasant, depending upon your spiritual preparation.

Lapis Lazuli

▶ **HARDNESS:** 5–5.5
▶ **COLORS:** A strong deep blue metamorphic rock with tiny crystals of iron pyrite and off-white patches or veins of calcite.
▶ **SOURCES:** The best quality of lapis lazuli has been mined in the province of Badakshan, Afghanistan, since long before Marco Polo visited the mines in 1271 C.E. It is also mined near Russia's Lake Baikal. A poorer quality of lapis comes from Chile, Siberia, Burma, Pakistan, Angola, Canada, and the U.S.
▶ **FACTS:** Lapis lazuli is not one distinct mineral, but a rock made up of several minerals. This is mostly blue lazurite mixed with smaller amounts of hauynite, sodalite, diopside, white streaks of calcite, and gold pyrite.

Lapis lazuli is often confused with azurite, a blue hydrated copper carbonate stone; the two stones often grow together. Stained jasper is sold under the name Swiss Lapis. Lapis has been used for centuries to make the color ultramarine for painters. The name lapis lazuli comes from the Persian word *lazard* or *lazuward* ("azure"), the Latin *lapis lazulus*, and the Arabic *azul*, all of which mean a very special deep blue color. Pliny the Elder said that the Romans called this stone *sapphirus.*

▶ **HISTORY AND FOLKLORE:** Lapis has been used as a decorative material from the earliest of times. It was prized by the cultures in Egypt, Mexico, India, Persia, and Mesopotamia. Excavations at Ur of the Chaldees turned up many fine lapis cylinder-seals. In fact, the Sumerians believed that carrying lapis was to carry the presence of a deity. The tomb of Queen Pu-abi (2500 B.C.E.) in the ancient city of Sumer yielded a number of pieces of gold and lapis jewelry. The Assyrian Moon god Sinn was portrayed with a long lapis beard, in proof of his great divinity.

Lapis lazuli was sacred to the Egyptian Great Goddess Isis, who was called "throne of the god" because she was portrayed with Horus in her lap.[30] This name also applied because she represented the divine royal wife, the marriage to whom gave each pharaoh his right to rule Egypt.

The Greeks and Romans rewarded those who performed feats of personal bravery with a piece of lapis. In China lapis was honored as one of the Seven Precious Things. Ornaments of lapis (*Liu-Li*) were worn during Chinese ceremonies in the Temple of Heaven. Catherine II of Russia decorated one room of her palace with lapis and amber.

The Assyrian word for lapis lazuli was *uknu*. However, many ancient Greek manuscripts refer to lapis as sapphire. Many historians now believe that the term "sapphire" in all ancient manuscripts should be read as lapis lazuli.

Physicians from ancient Egypt, Sumer, and Babylon used lapis for medicinal purposes, among which were relieving neuralgia and head pains, gallstones, depression, insomnia, fever, and curing eye cataracts. This stone was still being used in the late 1600s as a treatment for epilepsy, dementia, diseases of the spleen, melancholy, and nightmares, as well as to stop miscarriages. Today in Macedonia, women still wear lapis amulets, which they call the "stop stone," to prevent miscarriages.

The connection with the eye may have come from the use of lapis to fashion carvings of a stylized eye, which was called the eye of Isis or the All-Seeing Eye of the goddess Maat. Since Isis was said to watch over the dead on their final journey, this lapis eye was placed in the sarcophagus with the mummy. The chief justice of Egypt wore the eye of Maat when he rendered judgment. The Egyptians carved many objects out of lapis, including the scarab, the Eye of Horus, and the Heart. Small figures of the goddess Maat, goddess of truth, were also carved out of lapis and worn by judges as pendants; lapis lazuli was sacred to this goddess. The Egyptians thought so highly of lapis lazuli that they used great quantities of the stone for religious carvings of all kinds.

In the eighteenth century, lapis lazuli cost fifteen times the price of emeralds because it was so popular yet difficult to obtain.[31] During this time lapis was primarily worn as a strengthener for the heart and to dispel depression.[32]

Known to magicians as a stone of Venus, lapis lazuli was given as a gift to cement friendships.

Some writers connect this stone with the sign of Sagittarius.

Dreaming of lapis symbolizes a successful love affair.

▶ **HEALING ENERGIES:** A great healer and purifier, it affects the thyroid gland and the sixth, or throat, chakra. Although it helps one to see emotional issues more clearly, it will not calm down anyone who is overemotional. Helpful in treating fevers, epilepsy, and skin and spleen problems.

Excellent for healing and calming after childbirth, hysterectomy, menopause, abortion, rape, or abuse of any kind. Useful because this stone can remove painful memories from the astral body and aura.

▶ **MAGICAL POWERS:** A stone ruled by Jupiter, lapis lazuli aids vitality and virility by releasing tension and anxiety. Helps in balancing and cleansing all the chakras. Carry or wear a piece of lapis to attract a better job.

Increases mental clarity, creativity, and psychic abilities. Aids in communications with the Higher Self and spirit guides. Harmonizes the inner and outer selves by opening the throat chakra for greater expression and the release of emotions. Helps in overcoming depression. Used on the fifth and sixth chakras, lapis lazuli can strengthen psychic awareness and communication with higher spiritual beings.

MAGICAL USES

The energy of lapis lazuli is of a very high quality. This stone does not lower its power to your level; rather you must raise your mental, emotional, and spiritual energies to connect. It teaches you to set aside your personality and all its quirks, so that you can clearly see what is actually occurring within another person or any given situation. It will also wipe out any part of the past (either this life or others) that you are still carrying, but have no need to do so.

Lepidolite

▶ **HARDNESS:** 2.5–4

▶ **COLORS:** Pink through violet shades. Can be gray, yellow, or rich purple.

▶ **SOURCE:** Worldwide.

▶ **FACTS:** A type of mica, this stone is shiny and is made of layers of hexagonal plates. It also occurs in sparkling masses around pink tourmaline crystals. Because of its cleavage, as with mica, this stone is rarely faceted. Rich in lithium that gives lepidolite its color, this stone crumbles easily. Therefore, it is not advisable to wear or carry it, but rather to keep it for use on the altar or in the sacred space.

▶ **HISTORY AND FOLKLORE:** None that we know of under this name. A "new" stone to stone magicians, it is now being shaped into spheres and wands for use in healing and magic. Lepidolite is extremely fragile and breaks very easily.

Lepidolite is associated with Jupiter and Neptune.

To dream of this stone signifies that you need to balance your life by expanding your spiritual studies and awareness.

▶ **HEALING ENERGIES:** Soothing to the nerves; calming.

▶ **MAGICAL POWERS:** Creates harmony and connectedness with the Whole. Increases the desire to seek spiritually.

MAGICAL USES

Use as a focal point for meditations that involve regaining control of your life by mastering your emotions. It is also valuable to have nearby when studying spiritual issues. Calmness of spirit and emotions enables you to clearly understand ideas and issues you are unable to comprehend in a stressed state.

Lodestone

▶ **HARDNESS:** 5.5–6.5

▶ **COLORS:** An opaque iron black or gray black with a metallic luster on fresh surfaces.

▶ **SOURCE:** One of the world's largest deposits of lodestone is at Kiruna, Sweden.

▶ **FACTS:** Also known as magnetite because of its natural magnetism, this stone's name is sometimes incorrectly written as loadstone. The crystals have eight triangular sides. The massive and granular types of lodestone are hard, heavy substances that do not cleave easily. A type of iron ore, lodestone also is found in small quantities in meteorites and volcanic bombs.

The name lodestone may come from the Anglo-Saxon words *lad* ("a course"), *lithan* (to lead), and *stan.*

▶ **HISTORY AND FOLKLORE:** The Sanskrit word for lodestone was *chum-baka* ("the kisser"), while in China it was called *t' su shi* ("the loving stone"). The name lodestone may have been derived from "lead stone," because it was a directional finder.[33] This stone's other name, magnetite, probably came from the district where it was first recognized, Magnesia in ancient Thessaly.

The ancient Chinese made compasses out of lodestone as early as 2634 B.C.E., because of its natural magnetism. Many European seafarers have used magnetic compasses since the twelfth century; they also carried the lodestone as protection against shipwreck well into the Elizabethan era. Another use of this stone was to draw pieces of iron shrapnel from wounds.

The Greek Plato wrote that the name *magnetis* was given to this stone by the tragic poet Euripides, but that the more usual name was the Heraclean Stone. Lodestone was mined in Lydia, Magnesia, and Herakleia during the times of the Greek culture. Orpheus wrote that lodestone attracted the love of men and gods.

The ancient Orphic cult taught that if one sat in meditation and held the lodestone to the forehead, one could hear the voices of deities, see divine visions, and receive guidance.

An Arab legend about Alexander the Great states that he gave his soldiers pieces of lodestone, charmed to protect them against enchantments and evil spirits. The Mohammedans believe this stone protects against evil spirits.

Later, in the East Indies, it was the custom of one culture there for the king to sit on a huge lodestone at his coronation; by doing this, he was thought to attract power, riches, and favors. By the fourth century C.E., European men often put lodestone under their wives' pillows; this was supposed to keep them faithful.

The men in Mexico still carry lodestones in their belts to give them success and great virility. They regard this stone as a living being, every Friday placing it in water, then in the Sun, and giving it iron filings to "eat." However, they also believe this stone has a devil inside and will not enter a church with it. Another belief is that if the lodestone is rubbed on a knife blade, anyone wounded by that blade will die of the poison left there.

Lodestone was used to relieve pains in the hands and feet, help in childbirth, improve the memory, and repel enchantment.

Francis Barrett wrote that lodestone belongs to Saturn ascending and that it is believed to prolong life. Lodestone has been used in many attracting spells and to improve the memory. However, old records say it attracts lightning and should not be worn during thunderstorms.

Lodestone is associated with Gemini and Virgo.

If you dream of lodestone, it is a warning of subterfuge, double-dealing, and contention.

▶ **HEALING ENERGIES:** Used on one side of a body while other healing stones are held on the opposite side, lodestone is said to pull the healing energy through the body. For headaches, stroke the temples with a piece of lodestone. In Cornwall, England, lodestone is carried to cure sciatica. Also considered helpful in treating rheumatism, gout, neuralgia, cramp, and poor circulation in the legs. Stroke on the temples to relieve headaches and neuralgia.

▶ **MAGICAL POWERS:** Helps with communication with sea mammals, especially dolphins and whales. Ruled by Mars, carry lodestone to attract a favorable verdict in any legal matter or attract good luck with games of chance. Lodestone is also said to draw in money, love, and good fortune in general. Rub it on the closed eyelids to attract a lover; also used in certain charms to bring back a wandering love. Use to obtain a reality check and straightforward approach to any event.

Use this stone to align and activate the chakras, for it can balance both the physical and non-physical bodies.

Worn down through the centuries as an amulet, lodestone can be used to project the astral and mental bodies outward into space or across time.

MAGICAL USES

Since lodestone does have a magnetic quality, I do not recommend laying it anywhere near a computer or other sensitive piece of equipment.

Some healers recommend holding lodestone near achy joints to relieve the pain and stiffness. Others say that holding it to the temples or base of the skull will help to get rid of a headache.

Place this stone near the primary candle in a candle-burning ritual that is done to attract something. Excellent for money and love spells.

Malachite

▶ **HARDNESS:** 4

▶ **COLORS:** Medium to dark green with lighter green swirls and stripes.

▶ **SOURCE:** Worldwide, with Zaire as the largest and most important producer.

▶ **FACTS:** Found in copper mining districts, malachite is an opaque, green, massive stone, with its color coming from the copper. A stone with a characteristic bubbly look, malachite is cut and polished to show the alternating light and dark green layers.

▶ **HISTORY AND FOLKLORE:** The word malachite comes from the Greek word *malakhe*, which means the plant marshmallow, probably because of its color.

The ancient cultures of Egypt and Israel both mined large quantities of malachite as early as 4000 B.C.E. in the hills that rose between Suez and Sinai. The copper mines of King Solomon, located near Eilat on the Red Sea, also yielded this stone. The later Greeks and Romans highly prized malachite, making it into talismans. Columns in the temple of Diana at Ephesus were covered with malachite.

Malachite was used to make jewelry and ornaments, but the most popular common use was in cosmetics. Egyptian ladies used finely ground malachite to paint their eyes and eyelashes.

This stone was one of the prime gemstones used for power by the upper class in Egypt. The headdresses of pharaohs were often lined with malachite; this raised the ruler's vibrations to a higher level and opened him to wise counsel.

Ancient writers noted that the slaves who worked in the malachite-copper mines usually did not suffer from the plagues of cholera that often affected ancient Egypt. Thus malachite was often worn to repel plague diseases.

An old Russian legend says that anyone who drinks from a goblet made out of malachite will be given the power to understand the language of all animals.[34]

In later times, malachite was used primarily as architectural decoration, such as in the grand buildings of czarist Russia and the columns supporting St. Sophia in Istanbul.

A common feature of this green stone is the swirls of various greens that sometimes form an "eye" in the patterns. Sometimes called peacock stones, this particular pattern in the malachite was cut for jewelry or talismans to protect against the evil eye. Malachite was considered sacred to the goddess Juno, whose sacred bird was the peacock. A malachite "eye," cut in a triangular shape and edged with silver, was found in an Etruscan tomb. Malachite talismans are still popular in Italy. In some parts of Germany, malachite was believed to protect the wearer from falls and would warn of approaching danger by cracking.

During the seventeenth century, the power of malachite talismans was extended beyond protection from evil to include cure for all physical diseases. Finely ground and taken in milk, it was believed to prevent hernia, reduce pain during a heart attack, and cure colic. When mixed with honey and smeared over a wound, it was said to stop bleeding. Malachite amulets were worn by mothers to help with the teething of their children and to prevent convulsions. Many people used this stone to promote sleep. This stone is also believed to protect from lightning and contagious diseases, and draw true love and success. But the most prominent use of malachite was protection from all kinds of evil and enchantments. This stone is said to break into two pieces as a warning of danger.

Malachite is associated with Capricorn and Scorpio.

To dream of this stone means you have been blind to something or someone in your life that will cause you problems.

▶ **HEALING ENERGIES:** Strengthens the heart and circulatory system as well as the pineal and pituitary glands. Also revitalizes the body and mind and aids in tissue regeneration. Said to purify the blood as well as the spirit. Malachite has been used to treat cholera, colic, rheumatism, asthma, irregular menstruation, poor vision, and depression.

▶ **MAGICAL POWERS:** Malachite has a long tradition of repelling evil spirits, black magic, venomous creatures, and accidents. It has also been called the Sleep Stone because it helps with sleep.

An excellent balancer on all levels, it reveals and helps to remove subconscious blockages. Helps one to be tolerant and flexible to events. Opens communications between people. Stabilizes energy at a steady pace. Balances and heals all chakras.

Excellent for seafarers, explorers, and pilots. Also valuable for those who feel like they are at the end of their rope; however, you must take notice of your mood at the time of wearing this stone, for it amplifies whatever energy you project.

Very good for understanding the process of creating through magical manifestation. Helps to strengthen intuition and the power of transformation. Also raises the human vibrations so one becomes sensitive to the voice of spirit. Excellent for vision questing.

By strengthening the intuition and understanding, malachite can help you to move out of unwanted situations. Wear a heart-shaped malachite if you have been unlucky in love. When used with copper, malachite is said to attract love.

Put a piece in your purse or pocket to draw money, or carry with you to sales and business meetings.

Comparable to obsidian in many ways, malachite will become a psychic mirror during meditation, drawing you deep into other lives or worlds. It will uncover buried emotions and blocks that are connected to other lifetimes.

MAGICAL USES

Malachite has another magical power that is seldom listed in books. This stone acts as a mirror of the soul, reflecting only what is the true character of the person who uses or wears it. Therefore, it is best not to wear malachite when you are feeling negative.

Marble

▶ **HARDNESS:** 3

▶ **COLORS:** Generally light-colored background with swirls and bands of many colors.

▶ **SOURCE:** Many places around the world.

▶ **FACTS:** Marble is a calcitic and dolomitic limestone that has become crystalline because of heat and pressure within the Earth's surface. The finest marble is a pure white and comes from the Carrara quarries in Italy. Colors within marble are caused by veins and bands of impurities. Carbon, iron oxide, and other minerals create pink, gray, buff, red, green, and yellow marbleized patterns. Connemara marble comes from Ireland.

▶ **HISTORY AND FOLKLORE:** The ancient Greek sculptors used fine-grained white marbles from the island of Paros and from Pentilecus for their statues. Marble was also used for building great temples.

Marble is connected with the Moon and Cancer.

To dream of marble signifies a need of greater stability in your life.

▶ **HEALING ENERGIES:** Calming to the nerves and a busy mind.

▶ **MAGICAL POWERS:**

Black and brown: helps to focus energy on home and enterprise ambitions.

Connemara (green and black): enhances prosperity and feelings of contentment.

Cream and white: helps to focus on spiritual needs.

Green: prosperity.

Pink: calmness.

Salmon: helps to focus on the real causes of anger.

Tan: Creates a physical balance with the other bodies.

MAGICAL USES

One of the best uses for marble is as an altar top. You do not have to go to all the expense and time of covering the whole altar, however. You can simply use a marble tile or cutting board in the center, using its energy to recharge magical tools or power rituals and spellworkings.

Meteorite

▶ **HARDNESS:** 7

▶ **COLORS:** Usually black, brown, or tan.

▶ **SOURCE:** Outer space.

▶ **FACTS:** Meteorites are usually small pieces of alloyed metals or rocks that survive entering the Earth's atmosphere. The metallic meteorites are easily identified, as their density is nearly three times that of ordinary rocks. The stone-type meteorites generally shatter into many pieces upon impact; these tiny pieces are called tektites. Both kinds have a smooth dark surface that in time rusts or weathers away. However, an iron meteorite measuring 656 feet across created the huge Barringer crater in Arizona.

There are three main groups of meteorites: the irons (primarily nickel and iron); the chondrites (stone); and the rare achondrites (stone and olivine crystals). The most common meteorites are the chondrites. These are extremely old and usually contain minerals such as traces of olivine and pryoxenes. A few meteorites are what remains of comets and are composed of stony iron, silicate minerals, and a nickel-iron alloy.

When cut and polished, a metallic meteorite will show a pattern of lines and bands, something that is not produced naturally in rock here on Earth. One theory is that these patterns are the remnants of large crystals that were melted during entrance to the Earth's atmosphere. Their surfaces are uneven and rough, with a lumpy or scarred texture. Sometimes they have round or torpedo-shaped inclusions. Meteorites (tektites) do not contain the same crystallites as are found in Earth-formed obsidian.

Meteorites may be the remnants of disintegrating comets and/or asteroids. There are annual meteor showers, such as the Perseids from the constellation Perseus and the Leonids from Leo. At intervals of thirty-three years, however, there are intense meteor showers from Leo.

Small pieces of meteorite are sometimes called tektites; another name is melanotekite. The name tektite comes from the Greek *tektos* (melted). Although these fall around the world, they are more evident and recoverable in a belt that runs through Eastern Asia.

If you find or buy a piece of meteorite, or a tektite, keep it dry and preserve it with care to keep it from disintegrating from rust.

▶ HISTORY AND FOLKLORE: In Thailand, tektites are often carved and worn as a protection from evil. Meteor iron has always been highly valued around the world as the most magical metal available for special weapons and objects. Only special blacksmiths trained in magic worked this metal.

Meteors have also been looked upon as messages from the gods, signs of coming disasters. However, some large meteorites became parts of shrines. The goddess Ashtart's (also known as Astarte) shrine in the city of Byblos held such a sacred meteorite. Among the ancient Arabs, the goddess Al-Uzza was worshipped in the form of a large black meteorite. This is possibly the same black stone, the Ka'aba, now held sacred by the Moslems in the city of Mecca. The Ka'aba is marked with the sign of the yoni and covered with a veil.[35]

In more recent times, the falling of a meteorite, or shooting star as it is sometimes called, has become an omen of good luck. Upon seeing one, you should repeat the word "money" over and over until it disappears, or at least make a wish on it.

Meteorites can easily be associated with all zodiacal signs.

To dream of meteorite symbolizes an approaching event that disrupts your life.

► **HEALING ENERGIES:** Unknown.

► **MAGICAL POWERS:** Similar to obsidian, but with a denser energy pattern, it helps to reveal past lives and make contacts with extra-terrestrial energies by expanding the awareness.

Not a pretty stone, meteorites are fascinating and invoke inner visions of deep space and faraway universes.

MAGICAL USES

This is a very useful stone to use in meditations and/or rituals in which you are trying to connect with past lives. It is also valuable when astral traveling through the universe. Not only is meteorite a projective stone, in that it aids you in getting where you want to go in Otherworlds, it is also a base stone, in that it provides you with a sturdy, reliable link to the present physical.

Moldavite

► **HARDNESS:** 5

► **COLORS:** Dark olive green or bottle green.

► **SOURCE:** Moldau river in Czechoslovakia.

► **FACTS:** A deep green, silica-based meteorite which fell to Earth about 15 million years ago in the Czech Republic, moldavite can be confused with diopside because of its green coloring. This meteorite shattered upon impact, scattering small pieces of the mysterious green moldavite over a large area. The temperature required to melt moldavite tektite minerals into its glassy form is 200 degrees greater than that needed to fuse Pyrex glass.[36]

The first moldavite tektites were found in Czechoslovakia in 1787 and took their name from the region in which they were discovered. At one time, moldavite was thought to be volcanic glass; however, the chemical composition is decidedly different. Because of its bottle green color, it is sometimes called bottle stone or *bouteillenstein*.

A similar stone, australite, is found in Australia. It has the same effects as moldavite. The Australian aboriginals used these as charms for sickness and trouble. A few have been found in the state of Georgia and are called georgiaite.[37] Those found in Texas are named bediasites; those from Borneo, billitonites. A few others have been found in the Libyan desert; one such stone of 52 carats is in the British Museum. After a gigantic meteoric strike in June, 1908, an enormous crater in Siberia yielded similar stones.

▶ **HISTORY AND FOLKLORE:** One legend says that moldavite was the stone used to carve the Holy Grail.

Moldavite is connected with Uranus, Neptune, and Pluto.

To dream of this stone means a transforming experience will soon affect you.

▶ **HEALING ENERGIES:** Unknown.

▶ **MAGICAL POWERS:** Can balance and heal the body and mind. Helps when working with the Higher Self. Strengthens communications with other humans, interdimensional sources, and sea mammals.

A star-stone, moldavite helps when communicating with interdimensional energies and beings.

MAGICAL USES

Pair meteorite and tektite to enhance Otherworld communications and journey through meditation or astral travel.

Tektites

▶ **COLOR:** Usually black or dark brown.

▶ **SOURCE:** Outer space. They are often named after the country in which they are found. The majority of tektites are recovered in the Philippines and Thailand, although they are also found in the U.S., Australia, and Java.

▶ **FACTS:** Fragments of meteors, most often in small round or oblong shapes. The surface is usually rough from the rapid cooling of the bits of super-hot stone. Tektites look like dried prunes with many pits and wrinkles.

▶ **HISTORY AND FOLKLORE:** See Meteorites.

Tektites have the same astrological associations as meteorites.

To dream of tektites symbolizes the approach of a severe illness, either to you or someone close to you.

▶ **HEALING ENERGIES:** Unknown.

▶ **MAGICAL POWERS:** Said to help contact and communicate with extraterrestrials. [38] Balance the male and female energies. This stone can increase the energy field of any person or area.

Mica

▶ **HARDNESS:** 2.5–4

▶ **COLORS:** White to gray; many other colors.

▶ **SOURCE:** Worldwide.

▶ **FACTS:** Mica forms in sheets of silica that easily split away, and can be translucent to transparent with a glassy luster. White mica is known as muscovite. Minas Gerais in Brazil has mined large mica crystals; the largest measured thirteen feet across and weighed close to two tons. A black mica, known as biotite, contains large amounts of iron and magnesium; sometimes radioactive elements are also present.

Because of its fragileness and propensity to flake into thin, crumbly plates, mica is sold only in chunks.

▶ **HISTORY AND FOLKLORE:** None known.

Mica is associated with Mercury and Gemini.

To dream of mica symbolizes a need to organize your life or things will begin falling apart.

▶ **HEALING ENERGIES:** Unknown.

▶ **MAGICAL POWERS:** The reflective surface of mica not only provides a shiny surface for scrying; it also reflects back any harmful thoughts sent your way.

MAGICAL USES

In his *Encyclopedia of Crystal, Gem and Metal Magic,* Scott Cunningham gave a very useful description on how to scry with mica, or at least increase your psychic sensitivity.

Small chunks of mica set on windowsills will act much as the old witches' ball in reflecting back general negative vibrations.

Moldavite: see Meteorite

Moonstone

▶ **HARDNESS:** 6–6.5

▶ **COLORS:** White, gray-white, yellow, pale green, peach, brown, or pink with a blue or white sheen. Mostly or wholly transparent, this stone is primarily misty with a pale, shimmering reflection. Sometimes you can see an iridescence against its dark gray background.

▶ **SOURCES:** Worldwide, but the largest stones are found in Norway, Russia, the U.S., Canada, Kenya, India, and, Sri Lanka.

▶ **FACTS:** Other names for this stone are water opal, fish-eye, and wolf's-eye. A type of feldspar known as orthoclase, the moonstone is recovered from mines in Sri Lanka, Switzerland, and Burma. When cut along the cleavage planes and shaped *en cabochon*, this stone has almost a cat's-eye quality that changes with the light reflected from its surface. It is very rare to find moonstones of large size and fine quality.

▶ **HISTORY AND FOLKLORE:** Long considered to have connections with the Moon by all the ancient cultures familiar with this stone, moonstone was used during the waxing of the Moon for love charms and during the waning phase to foretell the future.

What we now call moonstone, Pliny referred to as *astrion*, *astriotes*, and *ceraunia*. He described these stones as being transparent, or nearly so, with a bright white spot that moved when the stone was turned, an apt description of an eye-stone. Pliny considered the *ceraunia* ("thunder stones") from Carmania to be the best kind; these had a bluish sheen. The Greeks also called this stone *Aphroselene*, a combination of the goddess names Aphrodite and Selene.[39] This stone has been discovered in Roman jewelry dating back to about 100 C.E., and in Oriental pieces even earlier.

During the Middle Ages, moonstone was worn by travelers for protection. It was also believed to grant success in love, luck in gambling, and a cure for epilepsy. The luckiest time to wear moonstone was thought to be on Monday, or Moon's Day as it was originally called.

Camilus Leonardus, a sixteenth-century physician, listed the moonstone as a selenite. However, selenite is an entirely different mineral. He wrote that moonstone contained the figure of the moon or a star.

The moonstone in India is a very sacred stone and is only displayed on a yellow cloth. They call moonstone *Candra Kanta* and say that moonlight of a Full Moon gives it occult and magical powers. They believe this stone brings great good fortune and enables one to see into the future.

In Asia, the best bluish moonstones are thought to be washed up by the tides only every twenty-one years when the Sun and Moon are in a particular relationship. As in India, Asian cultures look upon moonstones as very lucky.

The moonstone protects travelers, brings success and good fortune especially in love, and aids with mental inspiration.

This stone is often associated with the signs of Cancer, Libra, and Scorpio.

To dream of moonstone means travel and good health. It can also symbolize the unfolding of spiritual and psychic development.

▶ **HEALING ENERGIES:** Helps with female problems and childbirth. By unblocking the lymphatic system, it can heal and balance the stomach, pancreas, and pituitary gland. Can reduce swelling and excess body fluid.

▶ **MAGICAL POWERS:** Each person must work with the moonstone to see if it works better during the waxing or waning Moon for that person or the type of divination or farseeing one is doing. The moonstone is said to change its luster with the phases of the Moon, being brighter on a waxing or Full Moon and darker on a waning or New Moon.

Balances the emotions by reducing the tendency to overreact. Relieves stress and tension. Breaks up rigid attitudes and helps with emotional ties to the Higher Self. Helps one to see all the possibilities and discard tunnel vision.

Use during the waxing Moon as a love charm; during the waning Moon use it to foretell the future. Removes emotional blockages between lovers and helps to open communication.

Gives wealth and the gift of prophecy. Helps to make a connection with the feminine side of one's nature as well as with the Goddess. Works well with garnet. This stone reveals the truth behind illusions and will help to unmask hidden or secret enemies.

Enhances the psychic; helps to keep a piece with divinatory tools. For true seekers of higher spiritual development and wisdom, moonstone will open the gateway to the subconscious; at the same time this stone will not permit entry by those who are not ready for the experience. Aids in making communications with your guides easier. Use moonstone to recall past life spiritual experiences.

MAGICAL USES

If you are a sensitive person, avoid wearing moonstone during a Full Moon. You can become so open to the psychic and other realms of being that it can be unnerving.

Wear this stone when giving divinations and readings. Be prepared, though, to receive secret information that the person might not want discussed at any time.

A moonstone under your pillow will help you contact your spiritual teachers. This can result in waking up tired because you have been busy learning things all night.

Moonstone used as an altar decoration during spells will add subtle influence to the spell. Be sure you are not controlling someone this way.

Morganite

▶ **HARDNESS:** 7.5–8
▶ **COLORS:** Pink, rose, peach, violet.
▶ **SOURCES:** California, Madagascar, Brazil, the island of Elba, Mozambique, Namibia, Zimbabwe, and Pakistan.

▶ **FACTS:** This member of the beryl family was named after the late J. Pierpoint Morgan. It forms in short, stubby tabular prisms and is dichroic. The first morganite to be identified as a separate gemstone was found in California, where it was discovered along with tourmaline. It is not uncommon for morganite to have liquid-filled inclusions.

▶ **HISTORY AND FOLKLORE:** None known.

Morganite is connected with Venus and Scorpio.

To dream of this stone refers to an unhealthy attraction that could cause trouble.

▶ **HEALING ENERGIES:** Unknown.

▶ **MAGICAL POWERS:** Helps to heal prejudices and intolerance; creates a more flexible attitude. If you are attracted to someone who rebukes your interest, use morganite to break your useless feelings.

MAGICAL USES

If you are trying to break away from a relationship that is not to your best interests, wear morganite until you feel in control of your emotions again. This stone can also be used in candle-burning rituals for the same purpose.

Moss Agate: see Agate

Onyx

▶ **HARDNESS:** 7

▶ **COLORS:** May be brown and white, black and white, or solid black.

▶ **SOURCE:** Onyx is a type of chalcedony, which is a microcrystalline quartz. It is similar to agate, except that it has straight rather than curved bands of color.

▶ **FACTS:** The name onyx comes from the Greek word *onychos*, meaning a fingernail. One writer of the mid-seventeenth century recorded an old belief that onyx comes from the congealed sap of a tree called Onycha.

Mexican onyx is simply banded or streaked calcite, far too soft for jewelry. Such stones as Brazilian onyx, Algerian onyx, Yava onyx, cave onyx, and onyx marble are not actually onyx at all, but are erroneous names for stalagmitic calcite.[40]

Most black onyx today is not true onyx, but is instead gray agate treated to become a solid black color. This is accomplished by soaking the agate in a sugar solution for about a month and then heating it in sulfuric acid.

Gibraltar Stone is a variety of onyx marble with brown bands; it is found in the limestone caverns of Gibraltar.

▶ **HISTORY AND FOLKLORE:** Black agate has been used for at least 5000 years. At one time it was called nagel or nail stone. Early Egyptians learned the methods of staining onyx to improve or change its color. For centuries in the Middle East, this stone has been used as a worry stone because of the belief that it absorbs negative energy and relieves stress.

Onyx seals were very popular with the ancient Romans, who liked to use stones with different colored layers. Onyx was also used in inlay work, cameos, small sculptures, and beads. Originally, all cameos may have been amulets, for the word cameo appears to come from either the Arabic *chemeia* (a charm) or the Talmudic Hebrew *khemeia* (an amulet).

One English church used a healing onyx for years, even though it was engraved with the image of the Greek healer Asklepios (the Roman Aesculapius).[41]

One medieval Arabic text says that in China onyx was greatly feared by the miners; they immediately took it out of the country and sold it.[42] This may be the origin of the negative experiences onyx is sometimes said to produce.

At one time, onyx was worn around the neck to cool the sexual passions and to give spiritual strength and inspiration. However, the people of India and Persia still wear it to protect against the evil eye. In the Eastern countries, onyx is also used to counteract an ill-aspected North Node of the Moon.

One long-standing tradition about onyx is that this stone has an imprisoned demon inside it. This malevolent being is said to only be able to leave the stone at midnight. While inside the stone, however, this being must do the will of the wearer of the onyx.

Many cultures looked upon onyx as a stone of misfortune, which caused strife, miscarriage, contention between friends, and nightmares. This idea of malevolency may have arisen not only from the idea that it holds an imprisoned demon, but also from the fact that it is not advantageous for anyone with an afflicted Saturn to wear onyx.

Onyx is sometimes associated with Saturn and Earth and the sign of Leo.

To dream of onyx signifies a happy life with a suitable companion.

▶ **HEALING ENERGIES:** Use on present illnesses of the mind or body that have their origin in other lifetimes.

▶ **MAGICAL POWERS:** Ruled by both Saturn and the Earth, onyx helps in gaining emotional balance and self-control. Also balances the male and female polarities within each person.

As a Saturn stone, onyx helps with spiritual inspiration, resolving past life problems, and facing transformational challenges of this life. Protects against black magic and evil spirits. Helpful in recalling present and past life physical happenings.

Working with black onyx can aid in balancing karmic debts. It also opens the inner gates to listening to the voices of the deities.

Can reduce stress by strengthening self-control and bringing in good fortune and inspiration.

Black: helps one to feel secure and not worry so much. Can be used to deflect and destroy negative energy sent by others. Can also transmute these vibrations before a person is affected by them.

Green: calms and soothes emotions.

Orange to brown: enhances the personality.

Red: adds a dynamic quality to the personality.

White or cream: aids in creative projects by expanding the ideas and imagination.

MAGICAL USES

To most people the word onyx brings up the picture of a black stone. I happen to prefer black onyx, even if it is treated to turn that color. When I wear onyx, I am less affected by negative vibrations, particularly if I have to be out in a crowd. Black onyx will repel negative energy, leaving you feeling less vulnerable and nervous.

Sometimes, however, you will come across a piece of creamy white onyx, usually with a few traces of brown in it. This stone projects a soothing, dreamy quality that is great for relaxing and thinking.

Opal

▶ **HARDNESS:** 5.5–6.5

▶ **COLORS:** Precious opal is a light color with iridescent flashes; the black opal has a dark background. Common, or "potch," opal has no color flashes. Fire opal is a brilliant reddish orange; it is also known as girasol and Mexican fire opal.

▶ **SOURCES:** Australia, Czechoslovakia, the U.S., Brazil, Mexico, and Africa. Australia has been the main supplier of opals since the nineteenth century.

▶ **FACTS:** The opal is made up of tiny spheres of amorphous silica gel, which gives it its "fire" and play of colors. A non-crystalline stone, the opal can dry out and crack. A delicate stone, opal can have as much as thirty percent of its body weight in encapsulated water. This explains why too much heat can cause an opal to lose its luster, and why moving from a hot room to the cold outdoors will sometimes craze the surface, while too much pressure will cause cracks.

White precious opal can be white to light gray, dull yellow, light blue gray, or pale blue. The colors in its patches vary from violet to blue, green, yellow, orange to red. This stone is very brittle and will not withstand rough treatment. It has been mined for centuries in Czechoslovakia (the oldest opal mines in Europe), and is now mined in Australia, the United States, Mexico, Brazil, Japan, and Indonesia.

Water opal (hyalite) is completely clear but has a good play of color or "fire," while the variety known as hydrophane has no play of color until dropped into water or oil.

The fire opal can be transparent or semi-transparent; it is an intense yellow to scarlet red to orange shade that may or may not show "fire." Known to the Aztecs and primarily mined in Mexico today, the fire opal is one of the few opals faceted rather than cut *en cabochon*. Good quality fire opals are transparent, not milky, with a beautiful, rich orange body color. No other gemstone resembles the fire opal. It is also mined in Guatemala, Honduras, Australia, and the United States.

The true black precious opal is rare and extremely expensive; a stone the size of a small bean will easily bring $25,000. The black opal can vary in color from black to blue gray to smoke gray; its color patches are much the same as in the white precious opal. About 1887, in the White Cliff region of New South Wales, Australia, miners found several deposits of natural black opals. Before this, finds of natural black opal were very few, so unscrupulous gem sellers created them by dipping a light-colored opal into ink or allowing hot burnt oil to soak into the natural cracks in the stone. Australia is almost the exclusive supplier today of true black opal, although small quantities do come from Indonesia.

Other varieties of opal are moss, wood, liver, peacock, harlequin, boulder, and ironstone.

It is not uncommon for fossil shells, ammonites, and other fossilized remains to be replaced by precious opal.

▶ **HISTORY AND FOLKLORE:** One of the ancient Greek names for opal was *paederos*, which can mean both "child" and "favorite." The other Greek name was *keraunios* ("thunder stone"); a corresponding Roman name was *ceraunium*. The Greek and Roman name *paederos* also was applied to the amethyst and two species of plant, as well as to the opal. However, another Latin name for this stone was *opalus*. In Sanskrit writings, opal was called *upala*, or "precious stone."

To the Romans the opal was a stone of great good fortune and eagerly sought. When Senator Nonius refused to give up his very large opal, Mark Anthony banished him from Rome. The opal may have had some significance and connection with the Roman festival Opalia, an annual ritual to the goddess Ops. The Romans revered this stone as a powerful aid to prophecy.

However, the Russians took a totally different view of opal. They would finish no transaction or buy anything if they saw an opal among the offered goods.[43] They believed that any purchase in the presence of an opal would bring them nothing but bad luck.

In the fourteenth century, during the Middle Ages, opal was called the *Ophthalmius*, or Eye Stone; it was believed to strengthen the eyesight. This stone may also have been the Philosopher's Stone described by Arabian alchemists.[44]

The Norse *Edda* has a tale of Volund the Smith, who formed a very sacred stone called the *yarkastein* out of the eyes of children. The Brothers Grimm wrote that this Norse sacred stone was probably the milk white opal.

Albertus Magnus (1193–1280) wrote that there was a very large, magnificent opal set in the crown of the Holy Roman Emperors; this stone was said to watch over the royal family. This opal was described as a pure white, translucent gem that flashed with a brilliant red color. Called *Patronus Forum* ("Patron of Thieves"), this particular opal was believed to render its wearer invisible.

The idea that opals are unlucky may have originated from their fragility, although this stone was not considered unlucky, but lucky, in many ancient civilizations. However, it is more likely that Sir Walter Scott's novel *Anne of Geierstein* had a greater influence in branding the opal as unlucky, although Scott never calls the stone in his book an opal and the description does not fit. One of the earliest English descriptions of opal was written during the time of Queen Elizabeth I; nothing is mentioned about bad luck. However, it is still considered unlucky to have an opal in an engagement ring.

The Hungarian opal mines in Chernovtsy were very active during the Middle ages, producing great quantities of opal. When opal was discovered in Australia during the reign of Queen Victoria, the Queen quickly commissioned the Royal jewelers to make many beautiful pieces of opal jewelry for her, thus returning the gem to favor.

Ancient beliefs state that the opal can shield the wearer from any contagion and warn of poison by losing its color. If worn as a pendant, it was said to cure melancholy and eye disease, and also help blonde hair to keep its color. In ancient Greece, the opal was said to give the gift of prophecy. In India, they will pass an opal across the brow to clear the brain and strengthen the memory. Eastern cultures say this stone is sacred because it contains the spirit of truth. The black opal is highly prized as a luck stone.

Opal has been connected with the signs of Cancer, Libra, Pisces, and Scorpio. It is said to be ruled by Mercury.

Dreaming of opal symbolizes a happy, prosperous life. To dream of a fire opal means the arrival of money.

▶ **HEALING ENERGIES:** Soothes the eyes, heart, and nerves. Preserves health.

▶ **MAGICAL POWERS:** By stimulating the pineal and pituitary glands, the opal enhances the intuition and balances the emotions. Because of all the colors contained in this stone, it can be used to work on all the chakras.

Aids in making a conscious connection with the higher realms and the entities who live there. A strong prophetic stone that is easily programmed with either positive or negative vibrations, it is safer to buy your own than receive one from another person. Since opal brings up deeper past life memories, be certain you want to know about these before wearing an opal.

Strengthens the memory and helps to clear the mind; brings good fortune to business people, as well as promoting leadership.

Black: enhances sexual attractiveness; also leads one to higher spiritual experiences. One of the strongest good luck stones. Use with fluorite to clean the aura and prevent cording.

Blue: gives unusual creative ideas.

Fire, Sun, or Mexican: increases personal power and the ability to take action. Can break up any crystallization on any level. Helps to contact the Higher Self. Also attracts money.

Translucent white to yellow: clears energy blockages in preparation for new experiences; increases productivity. Carry or wear a white opal to attract money to you. A stone that can get right to the heart of a problem, it is not good for those who will not take responsibility or are too young.

White: increases productivity.

MAGICAL USES

If you cannot bring yourself to get rid of the bad luck idea surrounding the opal, then do not use this stone. Opal is extremely sensitive to the vibrations and mental energies of the wearer, projecting exactly the same vibrations that the wearer has. However, this is the very reason that opal is such a great manifestation stone. If you truly believe, for example, that your career will take off to new heights, your prosperity and/or spiritual levels will increase, or you will find a true love, the opal will beam those positive vibrations out, thus attracting just what you hold possible in your mind. Unfortunately, your negative vibrations will also be broadcast with just as much power. Do not use this stone if you are feeling pessimistic or down.

Pearl

▶ **HARDNESS:** 2.5–4.5
▶ **COLORS:** White, pink, brown, black; many shades.
▶ **SOURCES:** Persian Gulf, Indian Ocean, Red Sea, Polynesia, Australia, Japan, China, Scotland, Ireland, France, Austria, Germany, and the U.S.
▶ **FACTS:** Pearls, like amber and jet, are not actually stones, but hardened organic matter. However, they have a long history of being precious and used for magical purposes. Pearls are formed inside oysters (mollusks) when a piece of grit gets inside the shell; this action is automatically taken by the mollusk to ease the irritation.

The practice of deliberately inserting an irritant into oysters may have originated in China during the thirteenth century. After having a bead of mother-of-pearl inserted, the oysters were placed in wire cages and suspended in the sea beneath a special kind of raft. The pearls were harvested after three or four years. Very early pearl makers also inserted tiny wax images of the Buddha; when these were sufficiently coated with nacre they were sold in temples.

Three types of the small *Pinctada* oyster are commonly used to produce cultured pearls. Named after the color of the edge of their mantle, these are Silver Lip, Gold Lip, and Black Lip. The first produces white pearls, the second pink to yellowish, and the last black.

The great conch mollusk, found in the warm waters of the Gulf of California, produces a large, beautiful pink pearl that is patterned on the surface with flame markings.

Pearls are about two percent water and should not be stored in a very warm place or they can dry out and develop hairline cracks. Of all the organic gems, pearls are the most expensive. Pearls also decay and turn black after about a century and a half.[45]

▶ **HISTORY AND FOLKLORE:** The name pearl comes from the Latin *pilula*, which means a ball. Known since ancient times in the Orient, they were also valuable to the early Mediterranean cultures. The Romans consecrated pearls to the goddess Isis and wore them to attract her attention and favor. Mediterranean divers wore them as protection against sharks.

The term "cloth of gold" is mentioned in many ancient manuscripts, but does not refer to cloth woven of gold thread. Instead, this term actually means a cloth woven from an organic material produced by certain mollusks. Pearl-forming mollusks attach themselves to rocks by a bunch of coppery golden threads called *Byssus*. In ancient times, these threads were harvested and woven into what was called "cloth of gold."

There are many legends surrounding the origin of pearls. One, given by Pliny, says that pearls were created by drops of dew falling into open oyster shells at breeding time. This thought originated in the Orient where, it was said, at the Full Moon, drops of heavenly dew fell from the Moon and were caught by oysters; this dew then hardened into pearls. This may be why they also believed that pearls shone at night. People of Pliny's time also believed that lightning stopped the growth of pearls and thunder made the oysters miscarry. Ancient Arabian writers also believed this legend about pearls, but further stated that the oysters came to the surface of the sea only during April to catch the falling dewdrops.

In China, pearls were said to be the spittle of dragons, falling with the rain which dragons produce in the skies. Therefore, many

Chinese thought of the pearl as a talisman against fire. They also said the pearl would preserve the purity of the one who wore it.

Although the ancient Hindus knew that the pearl came from oysters, they also believed that on occasion pearls could be found in the stomach, forehead, or brain of elephants. Powerful talismans against all kinds of danger, pearls were associated with the Moon and therefore representative of lovers. Many traditional Hindu love potions contain finely powdered pearl.

The Scandinavian countries also have a tale about pearls and the god Baldur. When Baldur was slain by an arrow of mistletoe during a contest, his goddess-mother Frigg wept. Her tears congealed into pearls on the mistletoe.

During the Middle Ages, powdered pearl was added to antidotes for poisoning. Such medicine was even given to Charles VI of France in a fruitless attempt to restore his sanity. Physicians of the time believed pearl could cure vomiting of blood, hemorrhoids, excessive menstruation, and heart disease, as well as remove "evil spirits" from the mind. Burned with coral and then rubbed over the body, pearls were supposed to cure leprosy.

Finely ground pearl powder fortunately replaced the arsenic-laced face powder so widely used by the ladies of France and Britain; this was thought to improve the texture and luster of the skin. Ground pearls are still added to certain face powders and creams by the cosmetic industry today.

This stone is associated with Cancer, Gemini, and Pisces.

To dream of a pearl means many faithful friends.

▶ **HEALING ENERGIES:** Balances and heals all chakras. Helps in treating stomachaches, colds, bronchitis, and lung infections.

▶ **MAGICAL POWERS:** White pearls are said to be ruled by the Moon and Pisces, while black pearls are ruled by Saturn. The pearl helps in the search for higher wisdom and truth. It will absorb negative energy from anyone who wears it, then help that person to see and deal with the truth of self.

MAGICAL USES

I like to use single tiny pearls in connection with other stones. In this manner, the pearl will flush out the truth on any event, while the accompanying stone does its work.

I find that meditating on troublesome people or situations is likely to be clarified through use of the pearl. However, you will also be shown the truth of yourself and your actions regarding the same problem, so be prepared to face the truth and handle it. Saturn never lets you totally off the hook when it comes to responsibility. You may think you are avoiding the issue. Time will pass, and suddenly you will be facing a similar situation. This time you will not be allowed to evade the truth, and you will probably get slammed hard so you remember the lesson. It is just easier all the way around to deal with the unpleasantness the first time.

Peridot

- ▶ **HARDNESS:** 6.5–7
- ▶ **COLORS:** Olive or bottle green.
- ▶ **SOURCES:** Egypt, China, Myanmar, Brazil, Norway, Arizona, Hawaii (olive), Arizona (spring green), Australia, Burma, and South Africa.
- ▶ **FACTS:** Also known as olivine, the peridot has an oily luster and gets its coloration from iron. Although it resembles chrysolite, peridot's yellow-green spring color is much richer and deeper. The olive green stones are called olivine, the yellow ones chrysolite, and the spring green gems peridot. A few peridot show a deep green in dim light, earning them the name of Evening Emerald. Most commonly transparent with few inclusions, very large gems are rare.

  There is a rare form of peridot that is white; this is called boltonite.
- ▶ **HISTORY AND FOLKLORE:** People of ancient Egypt and the Mediterranean area got their peridot from the Jazirat Zabugat in the Red Sea. It was much prized and considered very sacred. The name in Arabic means "precious stone." At one time, peridot was more valuable than diamonds.

  The source of its name is not known for certain, and may be a corruption of an Oriental word for olivine. However, the gems that came from Jazirat Zabugat and were described by Pliny the Elder were known by the name *topazos* at that time. The island still supplies excellent olivines or peridots.

The Romans wore peridot for protection from enchantment and to ward off illusion and depression. During the Middle Ages, this stone was worn to gain foresight, inspiration, and eloquence. The peridot was often used in religious jewelry.

The Aztecs, Incas, Toltecs, and ancient Egyptians all used peridot to calm, purify, and balance the energy of the physical body.

Peridot has been associated with Virgo, Leo, Sagittarius, and Scorpio.

To dream of peridot signifies that you need to be cautious for a period of time.

▶ **HEALING ENERGIES:** A balancer of the glandular system, peridot helps with tissue regeneration and purifies the body by strengthening the blood. Most useful in healing spiritual diseases. Said to aid digestion and reduce fever.

▶ **MAGICAL POWERS:** A stone of Virgo and the Sun, peridot reduces stress, stimulates the mind, and amplifies intuitive awareness. Can balance and calm the emotions, as well as open up mental capabilities. Gives inspiration and strengthens the inner sight. Can aid in reducing jealousy and anger. Its stimulation for growth and change can be too intense for some; if this happens, wear it with amethyst or citrine to soften its effect.

By aligning the subtle bodies and increasing the desire for personal growth, it can lead one to new doors of opportunity. Can also help to discover your destiny or purpose in life. Opens one up to new adventures and challenges. Also said to ward off evil spirits.

MAGICAL USES

Peridot is indeed a spring stone, well beyond its spring color, as it has the ability to project you into a new life cycle. If you seem to be stuck and not moving forward, use peridot along with a white and a green candle. Place the peridot between the two candles on your altar. Light the candles. Close your eyes and visualize yourself before a closed door, a door that represents the changes and forward progress you want in your life. Visualize yourself opening that door, standing in the brilliant light that shines through it, and then walking into the light.

If you cannot open the door or become tired trying, extinguish the candles and try again another night. Sometimes you may have to practice this visualization for several days before you can get over the threshold. When you do go through the door, you may see something unexpected; not what you thought would be there at all.

Petrified Wood

▶ **HARDNESS:** 7
▶ **COLOR:** Many colors.
▶ **SOURCES:** Several places around the world. Biggest single deposit is in Arizona.
▶ **FACTS:** What we call petrified wood is actually fossilized wood. This fossilization occurs when all the organic matter is replaced over time by silica, which can be agate, opal, or pyrite. The wood structure is maintained, but the wood fibers are changed into stone.

The most famous concentration of petrified wood is in the Petrified Forest of Arizona.
▶ **HISTORY AND FOLKLORE:** Petrified wood was used by Native Americans as an amulet for protection from accidents, injuries, and infections. Widely used to ward off evil.

Petrified wood can be associated with any sign and is connected with the Earth element.

Dreams of petrified wood signal the need to do away with non-productive life patterns, relationships, or ideas.
▶ **HEALING ENERGIES:** Heals by building up reserves of physical strength. Helps to ease mental and emotional stress.
▶ **MAGICAL POWERS:** Gives the wearer a sense of security and takes away the worry about aging. Keeps the energy rate steady and attracts good luck. This stone can also erect an astral barrier that screens out and nullifies negative vibrations.

Use in recalling past lives or to read the Akashic records on the astral plane.

MAGICAL USES

I know one person who carries a piece of petrified wood on his key chain. He says he has not had any damage to his car since he placed it there. Before that, someone was always clipping and scraping his car in a parking lot. He considers it the best insurance he has ever had.

Use this organic stone in both meditation and while sleeping to tap into your Akashic, or past life, records.

Plasma

- ▶ **HARDNESS:** 7
- ▶ **COLOR:** A leek green stone; may have yellowish spots.
- ▶ **SOURCE:** Zimbabwe.
- ▶ **FACTS:** An opaque green form of chalcedony.
- ▶ **HISTORY AND FOLKLORE:** The Greeks called this stone *plasma*, meaning "an image." It was a favorite stone in ancient cultures, which carved and engraved it as talismans.

  Plasma is connected with Pisces.

  To dream of this stone symbolizes a need for stability in life. You have been lax in setting goals and following through with plans.
- ▶ **HEALING ENERGIES:** Unknown.
- ▶ **MAGICAL POWERS:** This stone can reinforce your will power, thus enabling you to keep on track and be more responsible.

MAGICAL USES

If you are a procrastinator or one who is lax about being responsible, carry a piece of plasma and touch it often. Let it remind you constantly that you have to make positive changes.

Pumice

▶ **COLORS:** Light gray or tan.

▶ **SOURCE:** Volcanic areas worldwide.

▶ **FACTS:** Pumice is a light-colored, porous volcanic rock that resembles a frothy substance. Its cellular structure is formed when volcanic steam and gases expand and explode as they reach the surface. It contains about 70 percent silica and 1–8 percent water. The finest quality pumice comes from the volcanic Lipari Islands near Sicily.

▶ **HISTORY AND FOLKLORE:** None known.

Pumice is associated with both the Earth and Fire elements.

To dream of pumice signifies a need to clean up something in your life.

▶ **HEALING ENERGIES:** Cunningham states that at one time women in childbirth were given pumice to hold, supposedly to ease the birth.

▶ **MAGICAL POWERS:** This very lightweight stone can be used to remove negatives from your life. It will also absorb negatives from the environment, thus acting as a protective agent.

MAGICAL USES

If you have had a particularly tense and trying day, breathe onto a small piece of pumice. Mentally see all the negative vibrations soaking into the porous stone. If you can, throw the stone into a body of water or a stream. If not, hold it under cold, running water for several minutes to cleanse it. This is a safe and easy method to use for children, who may be unhappy or angry about something.

Pyrite

▶ **HARDNESS:** 6.5

▶ **COLOR:** Brassy yellow.

▶ **SOURCE:** Worldwide.

▶ **FACTS:** The name pyrite comes from the Greek word *pyr* ("fire"); when struck with a metallic object, pyrite will produce sparks. This stone is also called fool's gold because its yellow glitter can be mistaken for real gold. It occurs in cubes with twelve faces, each with five edges, and has been used in jewelry for thousands of years. Archaeologists have found many such examples in the ancient civilizations of Greece, Rome, and the Incas.

Peacock pyrite, peacock copper, and chalcopyrite are all the same stone: pyrite with metallic peacock colors flashing over it.

True marcasite, sometimes called white pyrite, is a different mineral. Although marcasite has the same constituents as pyrite, it is an iron disulfide. Marcasite is also called the mirror stone. Since marcasite has a tendency to deteriorate over time and become coated with a white powder, however, it is no longer used in jewelry. Instead, faceted hematite is substituted today, although in a few cases pyrite is faceted and used.

▶ **HISTORY AND FOLKLORE:** Cultures in ancient Mexico made scrying mirrors out of pyrite; these mirrors were polished flat on one side (for scrying), while the rounded side was carved with mystical symbols.

Pyrite has frequently been found in ancient burial mounds, probably because it makes a spark when struck with metal, thus creating fire. Miners disliked the stone because it was known to cause mine fires when exposed to water and air; they called it *mundic*.

The French call pyrite by the name *Pierre de Sante*, meaning the "Stone of Health"; they say it affects the body's health.

Sometimes this stone is connected with the sign of Leo.

Dreams of pyrite warn that something or someone in your life is projecting an illusion and not the truth; find out what this is or you will suffer the consequences.

▶ **HEALING ENERGIES:** Corrects digestion and circulation by enhancing the blood.

▶ **MAGICAL POWERS:** Aids in harmonizing work situations and relationships. Strengthens the will and gives one a more positive outlook on life. Eases anxiety. Use with fluorite and calcite to stimulate the mind.

Can protect against negativity on all levels.

Iron: helps one feel comfortable with another person.

Peacock: helps one feel good about oneself. Creates a positive feeling if you and your life are different from those around you.

MAGICAL USES

To increase your self-esteem, write out two lists: one a list of all the positive things you are and do, the other a list of the negative. Place the negative list face down on your altar with pyrite and onyx on top of it. Place the positive list face up on the altar with peacock pyrite and crystal on it. Leave for three days.

On the third day have two metal bowls or cauldrons ready. Light a white candle. Read once more the negative list; then light it from the candle and drop it into a bowl. Say: "I release these. They are no longer a part of me." Read the positive list; then light it from the candle and drop it into the other bowl. Say: "I accept these and add to them. They are a vital part of me."

Flush the ashes of the negative list down the sink or toilet. Leave the other ashes in the bowl on the altar for another four days, then bury them outside or in a flowerpot.

Quartz Crystal

▶ **HARDNESS:** 7

▶ **COLORS:** Quartz crystal comes in colors other than the clear or white. The purple amethyst, the pink rose quartz, smoky quartz, aventurine, and the yellow citrine all belong to the quartz crystal family, as do several other stones. Rock crystal is colorless and transparent.

▶ **SOURCE:** Worldwide.

▶ **FACTS:** Natural rock crystal has some very unusual attributes. If subjected to heat, an electric charge is generated on its surface; this is called pyroelectric. An electric current is also generated if the crystal is put under strain; this is called piezoelectric. It is interesting to find these same attributes appearing in synthetic crystal. These qualities have made the quartz crystal valuable in the making of deep-sea diving instruments, clocks and watches, and the control of radio frequencies.

Sixty percent of the Earth's crust is made up of quartz, or silicon dioxide. Beaches are entirely formed of extremely tiny quartz crystals, dyed gold by the iron in the water.

Rock crystal quartz is divided into many categories. Milky quartz is white, composed primarily of encapsulated water and Iris quartz has an iridescence caused by numerous small cracks. Rutilated quartz contains golden needles of rutile, while sagenite (Venus hair or Thetis hair) has a net-like pattern of needles, which can be of rutile, black tourmaline, green actinolite, or epidote. Other types of quartz are individually listed within this chapter.

The largest quartz crystal on record is listed as twenty feet long.

▶ **HISTORY AND FOLKLORE:** Ancient peoples thought clear quartz crystal was petrified ice, formed in remote, cold mountain caves over long periods of time.[46] This belief was still held as late as 1777. Quartz crystal was in use by prehistoric humans in France, Switzerland, and Spain as long ago as 75,000 B.C.E.

The Greeks first gave the name *krystallos* or *crystallos* to crystal in general, and *acenteta* ("without a core") to the clear rock crystal. The word quartz may have derived from the Slavic *kwardy*, which means "hard." The first recording of the Latin *quarzum* comes from the sixteenth century, by the German writer Agricola; he said the Bohemian miners of Czechoslovakia used this term in reference to quartz. According to Webster, the English spelling was gradually changed from chrystal to crystal between the fifteenth and seventeenth centuries.

Archaeologists have discovered Egyptian and Babylonian crystal scarabs, vases, and cylinders, dating back to 1500 B.C.E. The Romans imported great quantities of rock crystal from Alabandina in Asia Minor, mostly leaving the stone unworked and unengraved. It became fashionable, though, for Roman ladies to carry crystal spheres to cool their hands during hot weather. The Roman armies also used crystal spheres and lenses as a focus for the Sun's rays to cauterize wounds taken in battle.

Also known as the Witch's Mirror and Star Stone (an old

British term), clear quartz crystal was used in many ancient rituals to start the sacred fire. The Greek Eleusinian Mysteries, held in honor of the goddess Demeter, started fire by focusing the Sun's rays through a crystal.

At one time the Ethiopian kings were said to be buried in tombs of pure crystal, which kept the body perfectly preserved. However, the Ethiopians were not the only ones to use crystal tombs for burial. In the city of Vienna, the Hapsburg family has an imperial vault in the Church of the Capuchins. Within this vault are 150 crystal vases, with a golden crown on the top of each. These vases hold the hearts of the members of the royal family. Duke Francis, who died in Switzerland, began this practice when he ordered that his heart be preserved and taken back to Vienna after his death.

During the 1800s, explorers found large quantities of beautifully crafted objects made from quartz in the French and Austrian Alps. These were remnants of much older civilizations, long forgotten up until that time.

The Irish Celts called rock crystals by the name of God Stones. They buried them with the dead, a custom similar to that practiced by some Native Americans.

Throughout Europe, Ireland, and England, a great many little balls of crystal set in metal bands have been discovered; these were probably common amulets at one time, worn as protection against ill-wishing. In some parts of Ireland today, these little crystal balls are believed to attract the favor of leprechauns and Nature spirits. Necklaces made of crystal beads were also worn for centuries by nursing mothers to ensure a steady flow of milk. Sometimes powdered crystal was mixed with honey and given to a nursing mother to increase her milk.

The use of the crystal ball for scrying can be traced back to the Druids. In Sir Walter Scott's time, these balls of crystal were still called "stones of power." To the Japanese, the crystal ball is known as *tama*; they use it as a symbol of eternity.[47]

From Medieval and Renaissance times onward, clear crystal was very popular with ceremonial magicians. Wands were topped with crystal points; crystal balls or points were used for contemplation, with the express purpose of opening the psychic mind; points were attached to a chain for dowsing or pendulum work.

Today clear quartz crystal is still used for divination and scrying purposes. Points, balls, and clusters are often placed on Wiccan altars for rituals because of the crystal's ability to amplify power during magic. Crystal points are often stored with divination tools to strengthen their power.

Early in medicine, the rock crystal burning glass was used in operations and the cauterizing of wounds. During the 1800s, doctors still used the old remedy of powdered crystal mixed in wine as treatment for dysentery, scrofula, glandular swelling, eye diseases, heart diseases, intestinal pains, to reduce fevers, and slake thirst. Crystal laid against the cheek was said to relieve toothache.

The use of crystal balls for foreseeing is well known. The use of rock crystal for scrying balls is very ancient and may have originated in Persia. However, until the mid-nineteenth century C.E., these balls in Europe were usually made of beryl, not crystal. Today, the Smithsonian Institute has on display a rock crystal sphere nearly 30 centimeters in diameter. The largest known ball of crystal was cut in China and was over 30 centimeters.

The Japanese call the crystal *tama* ("jewel of perfection") and have long used it to make crystal balls and beautiful art objects. They also call it the "breath of the white dragon." As *ching* to the Chinese, rock crystal has always been highly esteemed and regarded as a talisman of concentration.

The Arabs knew of quartz crystal and favored the rainbow quartz, calling it the iris stone. The iridescence of this type of crystal is caused by interior cracks, which reflect the light in rainbows. This type of crystal is sometimes called iris crystal.

In Australia, the Aboriginal medicine men say that rock crystal pebbles, which they call "ultunda stones," are embedded in their bodies to ensure magical and mystical powers. In both Australia and New Guinea, magicians use the crystal to produce rain. Certain Native Americans at one time regarded the rock crystal as a powerful hunting talisman and "fed" it on blood of the prey.

Some cultures of South America still believe that a spirit or the soul of one dead lives within each crystal; for this reason these very sacred stones should not be seen or used except by initiates. It is an extremely ancient belief that rock crystal holds all the knowledge and secrets that have ever existed. This may be the reason behind the South American belief that spirits live in crystals. It was worn to repel evil dreams and spells and to protect against enchantment, secret enemies, and poison.

Quartz crystal was used by the Mayas, pre-Aztecs, Aztecs, and Incas in religious ornaments and objects. The Mayans also used clear crystals to diagnose illnesses and treat them. The present-day natives of the Yucatan still dip a crystal into a bowl of rum, then scry by holding it to reflect the flame of a candle.[48]

The rock crystal has always been greatly valued in Scotland, where several of the clans have hereditary "victory stones." In some parts of both Scotland and Ireland, the people still pour water over certain ancient crystals, then give this water to their cattle as a protection against enchantment, illness, and attack by fairies.

Native American tribes knew about quartz crystals and used them in secret rituals for seeing into the future. They also utilized quartz for healing. Their shamans considered having a quartz crystal in their medicine bag a necessity to proving their shamanic ability.

Clear quartz crystals are extremely powerful stones and should be treated with respect. They have subtle effects on our bodies, minds, and spirits, which may be perceived differently by each individual. For thousands of years, crystals have been used to strengthen meditations and to develop the higher mind and soul.

Some writers do not believe in using leaded crystal. However, a few others, myself included, have determined that leaded crystals have the same qualities as natural quartz but much milder. Leaded crystals make excellent and beautiful pendulums and crystal balls. Their strength is very individual, so you must check each leaded crystal before purchase.

Unfortunately, this prejudice is also extended to polished and worked natural quartz crystal. As with lead crystal, this is an unwarranted dislike. Those who refuse to work with shaped and polished natural crystal are missing out on exciting experiences. For example, a damaged crystal that has had its point restored through shaping reacts by increasing its storage capacity and being better able to direct its stream of power with laser-like accuracy. I was gratified to discover that, years ago, the renowned crystal worker Marcel Vogel came to the same conclusions I did about the importance and power of shaped and polished natural crystal.[49] However, caution should be used as the shaped crystal can put out such a pinpoint line of power that it is easy to overdo a healing or spellworking until you are familiar with the tool.

Clear quartz can be associated with any zodiacal sign: for example, Herkimer with Sagittarius; rutilated with Taurus and Gemini; smoky with Capricorn and Sagittarius; tourmalinated with Libra.

To dream of crystal means freedom from enemies. It can also mean the unfolding of psychic gifts and prophetic powers.

▶ **HEALING ENERGIES:** An all-purpose healer that can be extremely powerful if not used with knowledge and care. Works well for any healing.

▶ **MAGICAL POWERS:** An emotional balancer, clear quartz crystal works on and enhances the pineal and pituitary glands and stimulates the thinking processes. It energizes all levels of consciousness. It also repels and destroys negative energies and vibrations, not only in the body's energy shield, but also in the surrounding environment.

Excellent for meditation as it enhances communications with the Higher Self, spirit guides, and interdimensional entities. Ruled by the Moon, meditating with a quartz crystal will deepen and intensify the meditation. Crystals set in a headband can help you with telepathy or aid you in gaining clarity of visualization; helps to enhance psychic powers.

This stone stores, transmits, and amplifies energy. Individual crystals can be programmed to hold certain energies.

Set at the four directions during ritual, or place with divinatory tools. Carry or wear a piece of clear quartz to change your luck.

Since clear quartz crystals can reflect every color in the rainbow, they can affect all the chakras at the same time.

Aqua Aura (clear quartz with a blue-tinted color caused by a very thin wash with gold): this stone has an intense laser-beam focus and effect. Will enhance whatever power is originally within the quartz crystal, or whatever power is programmed into it.

Double-Terminated: a crystal that has a termination or point on each end. Power can be drawn in by one end and projected by the other, or programmed power can be projected from both ends.

Single-Terminated: a crystal with a base or that is blunt on one end and a termination or point on the other. Energy is taken in from the base and projected from the pointed end.

Strawberry: redder than the rose quartz. Although it has an intense dreamy vibration, it keeps the astral body close to the physical body when sleeping.

MAGICAL USES

To clear, recharge, and ground a crystal, place it on a piece of pyrite or hematite. For a quick, temporary clearing, hold it under cool, running water for a few moments. If a crystal is particularly "dirty," cleanse it in a salt bath or burial as described in chapter 2.

Although some people like to set their crystals in direct sunlight, I have not found this a satisfactory method for myself, besides running the risk of cracking them or starting a fire. Instead, I set my stones in full moonlight, which seems to better charge them with psychic power. Crystals and other stones can also be charged, and their energy intensified, by holding in ocean waves, under a waterfall, or in a stream, as well as under cold running water from an ordinary faucet.

Bury a small piece or set around a plant to help with its growth. Place a chunk of quartz at each of the four property, house, or apartment corners for protection. If you are unable to place these crystal chunks outside, place them at the four corners inside.

Place a piece of clear quartz on your third eye while meditating on a question that concerns you; it will reveal images, symbols, or direct knowledge in answer to the question. You can also place a crystal at each of the four corners of the bathtub to charge the water and cleanse away all negatives, as Shirley MacLaine does.

Place four crystal points around your magic circle, one at each direction. Put a fifth point in the center.

When purchasing a crystal, do not be deterred from getting one with fractures and inclusions. Many of these internal fractures can look like ethereal doorways or miniature landscapes of another world. Some of the "veils" will also resemble clouds, gates, or temple veils.

For thousands of years, priests, mystics, and shamans have known that quartz crystals can aid in changing negative thoughts or conditions into positive ones, if the user is correctly motivated and centered.

Use incense made of sage, cedar needles, or sandalwood for cleansing a crystal.

To use a double-terminated quartz crystal for working with dreams, choose one that is at least 1 1/2 inches long and fairly clear. Hold it in both hands and think strongly of remembering and getting the correct interpretation of your dreams. Then place it under your pillow when you go to bed. In the morning hold the crystal to your third eye and ask the crystal to help you recall the dreams and come to the right interpretations.

Photographs of crystals, taken by Kirlian methods, are amazing. They reveal the crystal's energy pattern as a blue star-like center with radiations of brilliant white light. Each crystal will show a slightly different pattern of the radiating light.

Many famous people throughout history have used crystals as a source of inspiration for ideas. Thomas Edison called his crystals "dream crystals," carrying them with him at all times to stimulate ideas for his inventions. The French novelist George Sand and the English poet William Butler Yeats both used crystal for creative stimulation.

Rose Quartz

▶ **FACTS:** This type of quartz is light to strong pink, opaque to translucent, and somewhat brittle. It is also not especially plentiful, and comes mainly from Brazil, the U.S., and Madagascar. The rare transparent crystal found in Madagascar is called Rosaline. Rutile and star rose quartz are not common and are expensive.

▶ **HISTORY AND FOLKLORE:** According to archaeology, rose quartz was used by the Assyrians as early as 800–600 B.C.E. Later, it became popular among the Romans.

Rose quartz is associated with Taurus and Libra.

To dream of this color of quartz means a true love or friendship is coming.

▶ **HEALING ENERGIES:** A stone that heals emotional wounds, keep a piece by the bedside to release negative emotions during the night. Chakra blockages caused by strong emotions or stress tend to build up pressure and cause headaches, among other discomforts. Rose quartz will gently break up the blockages. It works well with amethyst. Can increase fertility.

▶ **MAGICAL POWERS:** Sometimes called the "love stone," it eases emotional and sexual imbalances, while helping to clear out stored anger, resentment, guilt, fear, and jealousy. Can aid in the development of compassion and love and is very useful in learning how to give and receive love. Can reduce stress and anxiety. Aids in creativity and building self-confidence. Enhances awareness of the true self; excellent for looking at who you really are. Helps in communicating with your spirit guides.

Primarily connected with the heart, or fifth, chakra, rose quartz is a comforting and healing stone, helping one to forgive and love oneself. One of the most basic of teaching stones, its greatest lesson is that if you cannot love yourself, you cannot love others. Also helps with intense grief if you have lost someone close. Can break up and remove painful memories.

Use on the heart chakra to reveal and bring to the surface buried negative childhood experiences, particularly those of great emotional stress.

MAGICAL USES

Rose quartz is excellent for use by children. Buy a large chunk for this purpose instead of a smaller polished stone, as small children have a tendency to put things into their mouths. The mere handling of the stone can have a calming effect, besides adding a vibration of warmth and security.

If seeking a true companion or lover, use rose quartz with pink candles in a candle-burning ritual. Rose quartz brings in a compatible person only, a friend-lover; it does not project sexual energy attractants. This is not to say you will not find a lover who enjoys sex when spelling with this stone. Sex will be only one of the features of the relationship, not the sum total of it.

Wear or carry rose quartz when you are despondent and need to feel loved and cared for. It is also comforting when you are sick.

Smoky Quartz

▶ **COLOR:** Dark grayish brown.

▶ **FACTS:** A clear quartz with a dark smoky color. Sometimes called smoky topaz (which is erroneous) and morion (a smoky quartz of an almost black color). Smoky quartz is actually clear quartz that has been naturally irradiated by the Earth. The colors of this form of quartz range from a weak tea-color off-white to a deep mink brown to almost black, and every shade in between. Smoky quartz is a discrimination stone; it helps to be selective in responding to people or events; and it cuts away dead wood from life. Use it with hematite to evaluate personal problems.

Although most smoky quartz comes from Brazil, very dark smoky quartz comes from Scotland and Colorado; Arkansas only produces clear quartz.

▶ **HISTORY AND FOLKLORE:** Before 3100 B.C.E., the Sumerians and Egyptians were using this stone. Later, it became popular among the Romans; many smoky quartz beads have been uncovered in Roman ruins. This stone was sacred to the Druids.

This color of quartz is known in Scotland as *cairngorm*, after the Cairngorm Mountains. There is a large smoky quartz (approximately 2 1/2 inches in diameter) in the tip of the Royal Scottish scepter. Cairngorm was set in the hilts of Scottish dirks and in brooches. One of Dr. Dee's shew-stones was said to be a beautiful ball of cairngorm crystal; this globe is now on display in the British Museum.

This color of quartz was also popular in the Western Hemisphere among the Navajo and other Native Americans.

In 1868, a huge cave holding thousands of pieces of rock crystal was discovered in the Swiss Alps. These crystals were all morion, a nearly black form of quartz. Several of these pieces are still on display at the museum in Bern, Switzerland.

When heated, smoky quartz loses its color and becomes clear. At one time Russian peasants baked smoky quartz in their bread to achieve this colorless state.

Not a negative stone, the smoky quartz slowly dissolves problems or illnesses. It connects with the Saturn qualities of stability and responsibility, yet helps to shift consciousness to higher levels.

Some writers connect this stone with the signs of Capricorn and Sagittarius. It is also associated with the element of Earth and the planet Saturn.

To dream of smoky quartz means that a time of stress and trouble is moving out of your life.

► **HEALING ENERGIES:** Found in clusters, double-terminated, and single points, smoky quartz can range in color from gray to almost black. It is very helpful in overcoming depression and severe mood swings and is mildly sedative and relaxing. Balances sexual energy; aids in fertility.

► **MAGICAL POWERS:** This color of quartz is excellent for meditation as it grounds and centers. It also breaks up subconscious blocks and negativity. A stone of discrimination, smoky quartz helps you to be firm about what you do and do not want; it aids in getting rid of unproductive people or parts of your life. Excellent for removing emotional blockages and the negativity they attract.

Strengthens dream awareness and channeling—a good stone for mystics and seers. Of great importance when channeling as this stone balances, grounds, and protects. It will absorb negativity from the aura and block out psychic attack. Also very good for linking with the Earth, its energies, and Nature spirits.

Morion or cairngorm, the very dark smoky quartz, is connected to the root chakra at the base of the spine. It helps with the instincts for survival and grounding on the physical plane; it also gives you the power and teaches you how to change your dreams into reality.

Dark smoky quartz can also force you to look at past lives that are impacting the present. Unlike other stones that only bring past problems to the surface, this stone will surface some and dissolve others. It has the power to break up the negative energy of those problems that one tends to hold onto long after payment has been made and lessons learned.

MAGICAL USES

The almost black smoky quartz can be set in various places around the house as a neutralizer of negative energies. As with the clear quartz, the smoky quartz can have doorways, phantoms, and rainbows. According to the energy of each crystal, they can be used for scrying, channeling information, or learning higher wisdom. Smoky quartz can also be set in the end of power rods.

Sometimes the power of smoky quartz is so intense that it is best used along with clear quartz to temper its intensity. Tests have revealed that a single smoky quartz crystal sometimes generates more energy than many clusters of clear quartz. Smoky quartz of this power and projection should be used only in cases that need extremely powerful stimulation.

Special Types of Quartz Crystals

Most of the crystals discussed in this section are crystal points that have various distinguishing features. These special features give the crystal points different magical powers or energies. The exception to having points are drusy, elestial, window, and some chunks of snow quartz, which are of a different formation and appearance. Most of these special crystals will be of the clear quartz variety; however, they can also be amethyst, smoky quartz, or citrine, unless a specific color-type is given.

Size of these crystals, as with other types of quartz crystals, has little bearing as to their strength and powers. Each crystal must be tested individually to determine the strength, regardless of its size. A quite small crystal can often be more powerful than a larger one of the same type.

Some crystal points will have multiple features, all within the same stone. An example would be an empathic crystal with a damaged point that also has the tiny figure of an animal or being inside it, making it also a teacher crystal.

Many times certain special features will appear after you have purchased a quartz crystal. Each crystal should be studied carefully over a long period of time. In this way, you not only become familiar and comfortable with the crystal, but you will also recognize any changes within it.

Channeling Crystal

▶ **FACTS:** The channeling crystal is sometimes called the Sage of the Crystal Clan, a spiritual growth crystal, or a seven-sided crystal. This crystal has seven lines or edges along the sides, which reach up to the slanted point. This termination slopes backward to a triangular point.

▶ **HEALING ENERGIES:** Since this type of crystal becomes so enmeshed with the vibrations of its user, it should never be used on another person. The only kind of healing possible with this crystal is that of the soul.

▶ **MAGICAL POWERS:** Aligns you with the Higher Self; creates stronger ties among the body, mind, and spirit, but on higher spiritual levels. Aids in making a connection with spirit guides and higher beings. Is an excellent energy shield if you truly seek a spiritual path.

Hold to your third eye with the point toward the top of your head. Ask to be shown the truth of a situation, event, or person, then watch for inner pictures or listen for inner answers. If you wish to ascertain knowledge of other stones, hold the channeling crystal to your third eye and the other stone in your receptive hand (the hand you do not use in writing).

The seven-sided crystal is an appropriate stone tool for the spiritual seeker or the mystic student, who is discovering her/his relationship with the Oneness of the universe. The number seven symbolizes the Goddess, hidden mystical knowledge, perfect order, and cycles in life. A channeling crystal becomes so attuned and meshed with its user that it should not be handled by anyone else.

Cosmic Crystal

▶ **FACTS:** Sometimes called a comet crystal. This crystal looks like any other quartz point, except that on one side are tiny indentations that look like a comet's tail, spraying out from a more or less leading head.

▶ **MAGICAL POWERS:** The cosmic crystal leads one on the path to an understanding of cosmic consciousness and its true meaning. Can activate natural psychic abilities and help with telepathy. Aids when one is faced with making a long-term decision during periods of transition or transformation. Stirs creative energies on all levels.

A first-rate energizer, the comet crystal will force the user out of the usual narrow little world of the self and open the heart and mind to the greater reality. This ordinarily happens swiftly, so you must be certain you want transformation before working with this crystal.

Crater Crystal

▶ **FACTS:** This type of crystal shows the growth places of smaller crystals at one time attached to it, but no longer present. These indentations can be either at the base or along one or more of its sides.

▶ **MAGICAL POWERS:** Excellent for anyone who must make sacrifices for the good of others, such as parents, teachers, caregivers, and the medical profession. Also very good for a person who has made useless sacrifices or one who has experienced "the bottom of the pit" and is ready to be healed of the emotional pain and trauma.

Creator Crystal

▶ **FACTS:** Sometimes called a baby within crystal. This crystal holds within itself a completely formed, tiny crystal. A rare formation, consider yourself extremely fortunate if you should find a creator crystal.

▶ **HEALING ENERGIES:** Good for working on infertility and successful adoption.

▶ **MAGICAL POWERS:** Considered a powerful shaman and dream stone, the creator crystal is excellent for use during meditation and with visualization techniques. Since this crystal does dramatically enhance psychic abilities and creativity, the user must be prepared for creative transformations. This type of crystal is one of the best for recalling past lives.

Crystal Clusters

▶ **FACTS:** This formation consists of a number of crystals all growing from a common base. The crystals can be pointing all directions or all upward. Most clusters will be of single points, perhaps with a very few double-terminated crystals. Each crystal within a cluster will have a distinct individual personality and power as well as working together with a group power. The size of the cluster, as with each individual crystal, has little to do with its abilities and strength. On occasion, a cluster will have a single or double-terminated crystal, either of the same kind or of another variety, growing in with the others, or lying across the cluster. If the crossed-stone is of a different variety, such as smoky quartz, it will add to and amplify the cluster's power, according to its abilities.

Crystal clusters can be amethyst, smoky quartz, or citrine, as well as clear quartz crystal.

▶ **MAGICAL POWERS:** Because the power from clusters tends to shoot out in all directions at once, a cluster is a natural cleanser of other stones and the environment in which it sits. Place the stone to be cleaned on top of the cluster and leave there for at least 24 hours. A cluster is also self-cleansing to a degree, although it can become overloaded with negative vibrations and will benefit from an occasional salt-water bath.

A cluster will also erect a shield against negative thought-forms and ill-wishing that may be incoming. Very good for raising the mood, consciousness, and psychic abilities of a group that works together often.

Devic Crystal

▶ **FACTS:** A devic crystal has a great many internal fractures and inclusions. They can be of any variety of quartz, any size, and sometimes have no termination points. The inclusions of water, gases, and air create beautiful interior veils, sometimes termed *fairy frost*. Legend says that fairies and other Nature spirits use these crystals as a safe dwelling place as they journey from one place to another. The original Sanskrit word *devi* meant goddess. Devic now refers to elves, fairies, and Nature spirits of all kinds.

▶ **MAGICAL POWERS:** This stone is excellent for establishing communications with Nature spirits of the elements, plants, and land itself. It also aids with telepathy and the development of the psychic. It can help heal sick plants.

Drusy Crystal

▶ **FACTS:** Drusy quartz is different from a geode. Although it is a quartz-lined rock cavity, the crystals inside it are very small and frequently rounded. In fact, it looks more like the inside matrix was dusted with infinitesimal baby stones. Druses can also be of other minerals besides quartz. Another name for drusy is sugar quartz, because the inside crystals do resemble a dusting of sugar.

▶ **MAGICAL POWERS:** Never a harsh stone, drusy adds a dreamy quality to spiritual and psychic experiences. A first-rate dream stone, it calms during meditation, while helping the user to awaken to self-exploration and spiritual growth. It is very good for working on manifestation or new cycles of life.

The drusy crystal works well with the geode as a personal recordkeeper, stimulator of creative ideas and energies, and protector.

Elestial Crystal

▶ **FACTS:** Also called skeletal crystal and smoky anhydrite, elestial crystal does not usually form points, but appears as an unattractive lump of stone. Often this quartz looks as if it has survived a fire; it has a smoky, burned, or gray appearance. It is also common to find hollows in it. Elestial crystal may have strange cryptic markings deep inside or on the surface. It is very different from any other type of quartz.

▶ **HEALING ENERGIES:** Opens emotions; releases emotional blockages and heals.

▶ **MAGICAL POWERS:** Good for anyone with a past history of abuse. Releases and heals emotional blockages; allows one to see the truth of the past as it is, deal with it, and release it.

Elestial aids you in understanding the path of this life by providing access to past life information that is still affecting you. This access and information becomes clearer and stronger when used with fluorite. An excellent power stone, elestial crystal can help you understand, deal with, and, if appropriate, break up old karmic emotional bonds. It is also valuable for astral traveling across time and space.

Empathic Crystal

▶ **FACTS:** An empathic crystal has had a hard life. It has been severely damaged, and its points are either broken or missing altogether. Many empathic crystals develop beautiful internal rainbows, a symbol that beauty and joy can come out of traumatic experiences.

▶ **HEALING ENERGIES:** A stone that balances the *yin/yang*, or female/male, energies, the empathic crystal can act as a superb rescue stone for anyone who has suffered abuse at any time. It is also good for working with depression, addictions, or simply long periods of life where you are inundated with frustration and disappointment.

▶ **MAGICAL POWERS:** The empathic crystal helps protect you when you are overwhelmed by the pain of someone else's problems. However, the crystal must be cleansed after being used for this purpose. It helps temper the feelings of loss, pain, grief, and fear that you, your family, or friends may be undergoing.

Generator Crystal

▶ **FACTS:** Also called a projector crystal, this stone's termination ends in six facets that come together in an almost perfect and centered point. The size can range from extremely small to so huge one could not lift it. Generators are always powerful and should be used with great respect. There have been instances where a generator crystal would crack other stones placed next to it, so be careful where you put such crystals. It is never a good idea to point a generator at anyone. However, they are excellent for cleansing and charging other stones, if caution is taken.

In fact, it is not good to leave any crystals too near computer equipment or storage disks or tapes. I did not believe crystals would do anything until my grandson stacked several crystals, points upward, on the shelf below my computer floppy disks. Two days of energy wiped all the disks clean.

▶ **MAGICAL POWERS:** Traditionally considered a shamanic stone, the generator crystal is excellent for concentrating and projecting energy. Although it can cleanse and re-energize all the chakras, it can be very harsh unless used for no longer than one minute on the whole chakra line. It can break up blockages in all the bodies. It is unequaled as both a channeling tool and a physical and psychic protector.

Use it in spellwork to focus and project energy into a project or for a manifestation.

A small generator crystal can be attached, point downward, to a chain and used as a pendulum.

God Crystal

▶ **FACTS:** Sometimes called an Osiris crystal, this stone is a dark smoky quartz generator crystal. It will usually be so dark that you cannot see through it. This type of crystal is a perfect companion for the Goddess crystal.

▶ **MAGICAL POWERS:** An excellent stone for releasing people or situations, the God crystal can make a direct link with the Higher Self and deity. It will support, aid, and protect you in all your endeavors, but only if they are of a high quality. It is an excellent energy cleanser, an aid in changing negative energy, moods, and subconscious thoughts into a positive channel. A shamanic stone, this crystal helps with dreams and soul rescues.

The God crystal can be used in ritual to represent the God energy of the universe, under any name that feels comfortable to you.

Goddess Crystal

▶ **FACTS:** Sometimes called an Isis crystal, this clear quartz stone has at least one five-sided face on its termination point. This is an excellent companion stone for the God crystal.

The crystal sphere, which represents a universal circle, is also a Goddess stone. The sphere has been used for thousands of years for scrying into the future, present, and past, all attributes connected to the Goddess.

▶ **HEALING ENERGIES:** Traditionally, this type of crystal is said to help with any problems concerning the female reproduction system.

▶ **MAGICAL POWERS:** A shamanic stone that aids with dreams and soul rescue, the Goddess crystal also helps in coping with grief and loss, as well as attracting and holding love. If used during meditation, it can aid you in remembering lost or scattered memories that may be important for your growth and/or transformation.

Guide Crystal

▶ **FACTS:** Sometimes called a dolphin crystal, this stone has a much smaller, shorter, perfectly formed crystal attached naturally to one of its sides.

▶ **MAGICAL POWERS:** The guide crystal is an excellent guide, just as its name says. Like the larger crystal directing the smaller one at its side, it can guide the user to the help and/or information she/he needs and into the path she/he needs to take.

This crystal can help you get in balance with the Water element, your emotions, and your intuitive nature. It also aids in healing emotional breakdowns and internal stresses of all kinds.

The guide crystal is a good choice in working on problems concerning your physical mother, any mother figure, or the Goddess as Mother.

If it is of smoky quartz, it can also aid in repelling nightmares.

Herkimer Diamond

▶ **FACTS:** Colorless, these small crystals were first discovered in Herkimer County, New York. Recently, however, a deposit was found in Mexico. They closely resemble diamonds, but are quartz crystals. Herkimer diamonds are clear and double-terminated. Unlike other quartz crystal, they do not form by growing out of a rock or inside a cavity, but instead form while floating free in soft clay. These crystals have the same double-pyramid shape as diamonds do.

They refract light internally, which enables you to see rainbows inside the stone.

Some writers associate Herkimers with the zodiacal sign of Sagittarius.

▶ **HEALING ENERGIES:** Helpful in diagnosing illnesses whose origin is in a past life.

▶ **MAGICAL POWERS:** More powerful than regular quartz crystal, Herkimer is excellent for vivid dreaming, remembering dreams, and enhancing the inner vision. Helps to relax the mind and body, thus avoiding stress by recognizing anxiety early. Also powerful for recalling past lives.

Able to produce and maintain a smooth, constant energy flow, the Herkimer will stimulate both the creative talents and psychic abilities. Excellent for prophetic dreaming, as it stimulates clear visions and allows clearer channels for telepathy. A shamanic stone, the Herkimer will also open communications with your spiritual teachers and guides.

It is not advisable to wear a Herkimer for long periods of time. It will draw you into a dream world and end up making you very nervous. Many people who are studying astral or dream work do well with a double-terminated crystal point or a Herkimer diamond.

Hydrolite Crystal

▶ **FACTS:** The hydrolites, or enhydros, are crystals containing drops of water. The crystal is usually cloudy, full of fractures, and is not ordinarily attractive. However, upon closer investigation, a small drop of liquid can be seen moving slightly in a tiny cavity inside the crystal. Never leave a hydrolite crystal in the sun or an overheated room, or the liquid inside may evaporate and disappear.

Some miners in California have died from drinking the water out of a hydrolite crystal.

▶ **MAGICAL POWERS:** The encapsulated water within rock crystal symbolizes the spirit within the physical human body and the various bodies that surround the physical human one. To some people, this drop of water, like the internal veils and fractures, symbolizes guardian angels or the ancestors. An excellent crystal for intensely personal work on the mental, emotional, and spiritual levels. Also valuable for making contact with Water elementals and water animals.

Meditate on and with a hydrolite crystal for better access to and development of the psychic abilities, particularly of a prophetic nature.

Library Crystals

▶ **FACTS:** A library crystal has a strange irregular formation of flat, stubby crystals attached to its sides. These attachments look like thick plaster, are merely slight rises, and do not have the typical crystalline shape.

▶ **MAGICAL POWERS:** Related to the recordkeeper crystals, the library crystal holds volumes of information—past, present, and future—within its structure. In some library crystals, this information also includes multidimensional information, as well as data from ancient cultures. An outstanding research tool, the library crystal is very useful in meditation for accessing past lives. It not only helps with any divination technique, but it can help you learn new methods.

Life-Path Crystal

▶ **FACTS:** These crystals are long and thin with one or more absolutely smooth sides. This smoothness can often only be detected by rubbing a finger down the sides of the stone. Sometimes called beautyway crystals, these are not common and difficult to find. The power of this type of crystal is augmented when it is used with sugilite.

▶ **MAGICAL POWERS:** A strong shamanic stone, the life-path crystal is excellent for protection, fighting depression, and working with divination. It will activate and empower any latent psychic abilities and intuitional energies. This crystal is excellent for making contact with teachers and guides. If used during meditation and spiritual studies, it will help you discover and maintain the planned purpose with which you came into this life.

Although the life-path crystal works well on spiritual pursuits, it will also aid in business, career, or entrepreneurial goals. It aids in determining what is important for your life and helps in discarding the unnecessary things.

Master Programmer Crystal

▶ **FACTS:** Sometimes called a master matrix or a root directory crystal, master programmer will have most, if not all, of the known geometric symbols naturally etched either on its sides or buried within it. These are extremely rare and can be any variety of crystal. They are not an especially beautiful crystal, but are so powerful that misusing one will give you a violent headache.

▶ **MAGICAL POWERS:** The master programmer cannot be programmed itself. It can, however, reprogram the recordkeeper crystal if its data becomes damaged or lost. It contains all information available to humans at the present time. Used with the library crystal, the master programmer will strengthen the contact with that stone, allowing you greater access to ancient esoteric knowledge. It is also very good for making contact with your teachers and guides.

Matriarch Crystal

▶ **FACTS:** Sometimes called a barnacle crystal, this stone will be encrusted along one of its sides with new, smaller, stubby crystals.

▶ **MAGICAL POWERS:** Like a wise, well-loved family matriarch, this type of crystal is valuable in healing family and community difficulties. It also helps with any kind of issue that affects the well-being of women and children. A crystal of strong feminine vibrations, Matriarch can help both men and women get in touch with their feminine energies and become better-integrated personalities.

Moon Crystal

▶ **FACTS:** Also called a Selene crystal (after the Greek goddess of the Moon), this stone has within it a rounded inclusion that resembles a phase of the Moon. This can be a complete circle, a semi-circle, or a small sliver rounded on one side.

▶ **MAGICAL POWERS:** A representative of all Moon deities, this crystal becomes highly charged during any Full Moon. It will stimulate natural psychic and intuitive abilities, while providing insight into esoteric mysteries. Because the Moon crystal can help control and neutralize anger and frustration, it is an excellent balance stone for physical activity, emotions, mental pursuits, and spiritual endeavors. If properly accessed during the Full Moon, this crystal will also enhance creativity to a high degree.

Muse Crystal

▶ **FACTS:** This type of crystal has nine completely formed crystal points, all of similar size and length, naturally attached to each other. Breaking nine stones out of a larger cluster does not make a muse crystal. A rare formation, this type of crystal is also known as a triple quantum.

▶ **MAGICAL POWERS:** One of the best stones available for divination and creative expression, the muse crystal will greatly intensify the psychic and access to the subconscious mind. If you have had past lives in psychic or creative pursuits, this crystal will bring these latent abilities to the fore. A symbol of the Nine-Fold Goddess, the muse crystal is absolutely the best there is for anyone engaged in any type of creative endeavor.

Parent Crystal

▶ **FACTS:** Sometimes called an inner-child or in-and-out crystal, one form of this stone has one or more smaller crystals partially embedded inside it and projecting from its sides. Another form is a small crystal attached between two larger crystals.

▶ **MAGICAL POWERS:** This crystal is very valuable as an aid for any kind of manifestation. It teaches hope and patience when working toward a future goal.

The parent crystal can aid in uncovering the truth behind past or present child-parent problems by cutting through all illusions and showing the truth. Sometimes this can be difficult and very emotional, but the benefits are positive. When the truth is faced and accepted, this crystal will slowly absorb the emotional traumas associated with the situation. It will put you back on track concerning what you came here to learn, especially from the difficult situations.

A valuable emotional and physical protector, this crystal helps release stress and depression. It aids in the interpretation of dreams and can even cause intense dreaming as a method of solving problems.

Phantom Quartz

▶ **FACTS:** A phantom crystal is a crystal that has within it the ghostly, shadowy outlines of other crystal formations. It looks as if one crystal or pyramid has grown over the top of another or several others. These inner shadowy crystals are not fully formed; usually only ghosts of the terminated ends are seen and there are no hard outlines. Phantom crystals can be found in many colors and shapes, but are not common.

▶ **HEALING ENERGIES:** An excellent stone for children to learn meditation, the phantom crystal also works well on children's illnesses, or adult's illnesses that stem from something in childhood.

▶ **MAGICAL POWERS:** A strong shamanic stone, this crystal works well when tracing past lives as far back as you wish to go; it works during both meditation and sleep. It is excellent to use during periods of great transition, as it releases stress and intensifies psychic awareness. It will protect and shield while stimulating creativity and growth. Its protection qualities help with understanding and dealing with grief and loss.

Planet Crystal

▶ **FACTS:** This crystal is most unusual in that it is generally a clear quartz crystal that has a layer of the rock matrix still attached at its base or along one side. When looking through the crystal, one sees what appears to be an aerial view of a planet. The matrix looks like mountains, trees, and deserts far below.

▶ **HEALING ENERGIES:** This strange crystal can be used to heal the Earth.

▶ **MAGICAL POWERS:** A powerful, but gentle, stone, the planet crystal can aid in astral travel to other universes and across time and space. It works well with other crystals that have the same attributes.

Prosperity Crystal

▶ **FACTS:** Sometimes called an abundance crystal, this type of crystal has a number of very small, perfectly formed crystals clustered around its base or attached to its sides. It can be any color and variety of crystal.

▶ **MAGICAL POWERS:** A symbol that you can create what you want and need in your life, the prosperity crystal magnifies and manifests what you truly believe you deserve. Therefore, be certain you are in a positive mood and have clear positive ideas of abundance when you use this crystal. Excellent for anyone, but especially for those who are business/career-oriented.

If you do not feel positive toward abundance, work with this crystal to replace those feelings with positive ones. Even when you become more positive, working with a prosperity crystal will give you unlimited potential for growth.

This is also an excellent stone for anyone who is taking back her/his personal power after a negative happening in life. Especially good for those who are recovering from a physical trauma, financial disaster, or negative relationship.

Rainbow Crystal

▶ **FACTS:** A crystal with inclusions of water or another mineral that reflects the colors of the rainbow when the stone is turned in the light. Also called iris quartz, a good quality rainbow crystal is much rarer than diamonds and can be very expensive. Although rainbows can be found in other varieties of quartz, they are most spectacular in the clear quartz.

▶ **HEALING ENERGIES:** A powerful rescue stone, the rainbow crystal primarily works on healing emotional damage and pain.

▶ **MAGICAL POWERS:** Excellent for survivors of any trauma, physical or emotional. The rainbow will help you fight against depression and despair, gain optimism and hope for the future, and find happiness. It can even strengthen protection for you during difficult times. A crystal that has strong connections between this world and the astral world, the rainbow crystal is very good when astral traveling.

Receiver-Generator Crystal

▶ **FACTS:** This type of crystal is a generator crystal that has one face of its point sloping inward more than the other five faces. The facets of its point do not come to a perfectly centered end.

▶ **MAGICAL POWERS:** A crystal that simultaneously receives and projects energy patterns, the receiver-generator will cleanse and recharge anything—humans, animals, plants, or other stones. This type of crystal will aid in creating transformations and strengthening your ability to communicate with those in both this world and the astral world. It is excellent for divination and telepathy.

Recordkeeper Crystal

▶ **FACTS:** Sometimes called a recorder crystal, this stone has a geometric symbol naturally etched into one or more of its sides or point-facets. Usually this symbol is a triangle. These symbols may be visible only under a strong light. Other times you can feel the pattern of these symbols when you run your finger over the sides of the crystal.

It is said that the information stored in recordkeeper crystals can only be accessed when you match your vibrational level with that of the stone. Recordkeeper crystals have also been known to disappear if the custodian (which is all you can ever be of such a crystal) is careless or disrespectful of its usage. A powerful stone, this crystal should be treated with great respect and care.

▶ **MAGICAL POWERS:** Outstanding as a dream and meditation stone, the recordkeeper crystal aids in accessing ancient information and records. It also helps you gain knowledge of past-life memories. If you are engaged in development of the psychic, particularly in the area of divination, this crystal will add to your spiritual growth and power.

Rutilated Quartz

▶ **FACTS:** Rutilated quartz is clear rock crystal containing thin threads of gold or titanium, or such other penetrating minerals as asbestos and actinolite inside it.

▶ **HISTORY AND FOLKLORE:** This type of crystal is known to the French as *fleches d'amour*, or "love's arrows"; they are also called Venus's hair stone, Thetis's hair stone, pencils of Venus, Cupid's arrows, Cupid's net, or the Goddess's tresses.

The rutiles augment the transmission power and energy of the quartz. If the rutiles are silver, the energy is of a gentler nature; if the rutiles are gold or reddish, the energy is more intense.

Rutilated quartz has been connected to the signs of Gemini and Taurus.

▶ **HEALING ENERGIES:** A very powerful healer stone, rutilated quartz is harder to control and send with than clear crystal; it takes much patience and work with the self before control over its energy can be established.

It affects all the chakras and can regenerate damaged tissue. Can also repel or dissolve depression. Excellent for balancing and healing on all levels. Use with beryl to help bronchitis and asthma. A general detoxifying stone, rutilated quartz is good for drug or smoking problems.

▶ **MAGICAL POWERS:** By enhancing the life-force energy, rutilated crystal strengthens the immune system and stimulates the thinking processes. A highly electric stone, denser than ordinary clear crystal, it can increase clairvoyance by piercing through layers of physical, emotional, and mental density. It transmutes negative energy, thus helping with communication with the Higher Self and spirit guides. Enables one to project an aura of power and authority, while keeping the perspective very clear.

Rutile adds power to whatever stone it is in. It magnifies the user's personal aura, giving an aura of authority and clarity in power.

A good energy stone, rutilated quartz will increase the efficiency of magic if worn or placed on the altar during rituals.

Combining the powers of both rutile and clear quartz, this stone strengthens insight and the understanding of problems.

Smoky quartz: can help to balance the chakras and bring on prophetic dreaming. It also aids in calming fears and easing depression.

Venus hair: excellent for meditation on the Goddess. Especially beautiful when the light falls on the rutile needles in this stone, one can be drawn deeply into meditation by the glitter.

Scepter Crystal

▶ **FACTS:** This type of crystal is an ordinary quartz crystal with a cap overgrowing its pointed end. This cap is a new crystal that grew on top of the older one. The crystals can range in size from 1/4 inch to several inches in length and can be any color or variety of crystal.

▶ **MAGICAL POWERS:** A symbol of the power of the Goddess and God, the scepter crystal is excellent for channeling and communicating with your teachers and guides. A generator of psychic energy, this stone can make you aware of all that goes on around you, both externally and internally. The scepter crystal can also stimulate you to take positive action and follow through with it.

The scepter crystal adds a note of personal power for any magician, priestess, or priest who uses it during the performance of a ritual.

Singing Crystal

▶ **FACTS:** Also called a toning crystal, this stone is usually long, thin, and of perfectly clear quartz crystal. The angles are so sharp and straight that they might appear to be manmade. Infrequently, singing crystals may have small side projections off the main crystal.

The singing crystal produces a pleasant tone when struck gently with another crystal. When held during chanting, you will feel sympathetic vibrations resonating from the stone. These crystals are used primarily to amplify singing, chanting, speaking, or musical sounds. They can also be used to store the energy vibrations of these sounds.

▶ **HEALING ENERGIES:** Use when chanting during healings to intensify the healing energies.

▶ **MAGICAL POWERS:** This is an excellent choice when learning the magic of sound and light. It is outstanding for meditation and astral travel where you are using the vibrations of sound to aid you. It can also build a psychic bridge between the Earth and other planets in the universe.

Snow Quartz

▶ **FACTS:** A cloudy, white form of quartz found in the U.S., Brazil, Alaska, and Mexico, the appearance of this stone is caused by trapped inclusions of gases, air, and water that make it opaque, cloudy, and snow-like. This crystal is also called milky quartz. The snow quartz may come in either points or chunks.

▶ **MAGICAL POWERS:** Use to gain clear insights and free the user of cynicism; it is very good for children. By activating the crown chakra, this stone can help with the development of psychic abilities. An observation stone, it provides fresh, clear insights.

Soul Mate Crystal

▶ **FACTS:** A soul mate crystal is composed of two crystals growing naturally side by side. They will be of equal length and size. The pair does not have to be perfectly aligned top and bottom. Usually, these are single-terminated.

▶ **MAGICAL POWERS:** This crystal is an excellent choice for meditation and dreaming as it connects you with the various aspects of your personality, integrating them into a positive, smooth-working whole. It can also connect you with past lives that are influencing your present life, thus enabling you to see and deal with any carry-over negatives.

This paired crystal will also attract soul mates, although one should be very careful in using it for this purpose. One who was an agreeable soul mate in another life may have evolved into a person with whom you have little in common this time.

Spirit Guardian Crystal

▶ **FACTS:** A spirit guardian crystal must be two double-terminated crystals attached naturally on the side. The crystals will be of equal or nearly equal length.

▶ **MAGICAL POWERS:** These are very personal crystals. If you are fortunate enough to find a spirit guardian crystal, treat it with respect and care. It is one of the most powerful stones for connecting you with your spiritual teachers, guides, and guardians. It is also one of the most powerful protection crystals to use when astral traveling or meditating.

The spirit guardian crystal helps you to find and correctly understand ancient, forgotten knowledge.

Tabular Crystal

▶ **FACTS:** Sometimes called "tabbies," these crystals are of a flattened tabular shape. This means that two of the opposing sides will be twice as wide or more than the other sides. They may or may not have a termination point.

▶ **HEALING ENERGIES:** Because of the tabular crystal's ability to connect all types of energies, it can be a valuable tool in healing. It will create a smooth-flowing connection between all the chakras.

▶ **MAGICAL POWERS:** Because of its powerful bridging energy, the tabular crystal can create a useful path between the conscious and subconscious minds. Excellent for channeling, it will also project a safe area of calm and relaxation. It can also be used to bridge or connect the power of other gemstones.

The energy coming from a tabular crystal will be of a different frequency than other crystal formations.

Teacher Crystals

▶ **FACTS:** Usually a quartz crystal with great beauty and light, the teacher crystal will hold, deep within it, the tiny form of an animal or human-like being. Some have more than one such figure. The figures within this type of crystal have been known to change into something completely different over time.

▶ **MAGICAL POWERS:** This specific type of quartz crystal is said to hold great amounts of knowledge. It is believed that teacher crystals appear when the student is ready, that one does not go out seeking and finding them. It is also said that one will not be allowed to unlock the stored knowledge of this crystal until one is ready to assimilate the information.

A powerful shamanic and dream stone, the teacher crystal will stimulate psychic development and activate important teaching dreams. It strengthens divination and boosts creativity. This type of crystal also creates better communications with your teachers and guides.

Time-Link Crystal

▶ **FACTS:** This type of crystal will have a parallelogram on one of the faces of its point. A parallelogram, according to *Webster's Dictionary*, is a quadrilateral form with opposite sides parallel and equal in length.

▶ **MAGICAL POWERS:** This crystal has the power to work both inside and outside of time's limitations, thus making it possible for you to access the past, present, and future. It is valuable in recalling past lives or seeing into the future through dreams and channeling.

Time-Travel Crystal

▶ **FACTS:** Sometimes called a mythic crystal, this crystal is a double-terminated snow quartz stone. Although this crystal is ordinarily opaque because of the large amounts of trapped air, gas, and water inside it, it can have tiny clear spaces.

▶ **MAGICAL POWERS:** Outstanding for use in meditation, this crystal enables you to move backward and forward through time in Earth's history. It stimulates spiritual balance as well as personal creativity.

Tourmalinated Quartz

▶ **FACTS:** Clear quartz with black tourmaline crystals suspended inside. Wolframite quartz is black tablets of this mineral found in quartz. Tourmalinated quartz is considered to have double the power of clear crystal. The black tourmaline works to balance opposites in energy.

Some writers associated this stone with the sign of Libra.

▶ **HEALING ENERGIES:** Realigns and balances the aura. Helps to let go of any old conditions that are destructive to a positive future and are having an adverse physical effect. Helps with depression and nervous exhaustion.

▶ **MAGICAL POWERS:** Combines the vibrational powers of the clear crystal and the black tourmaline. Balances all extremes as well as the male and female polarities. A grounding stone, it is also very protective and breaks up negativity. Helps in eliminating negative conditioning. Use during ritual to balance contrasting elements.

Quartz with black wolframite tablets brings in new karmas and begins new cycles.

Triple Crystal

▶ **FACTS:** Sometimes called a quantum crystal, this is a natural cluster of three single-terminated crystals attached to one another at the sides or the base. This must be a natural formation, not broken out of another cluster. The crystals must be equal, or nearly so, in size and length. The power of rare double-terminated triple crystals is vastly increased.

▶ **MAGICAL POWERS:** A symbol of the Triple Goddess, this stone should be used with caution, as it is one of the most potent of the crystals. An outstanding shamanic and dream crystal, the triple boosts psychic energy and transformation. Be very certain of all your true reasons for wanting something before you use this crystal to get it. If your reasons and emotions are unclear or negative, the energy could well rebound upon you in a devastating fashion. Excellent to use when trying to end a conflict.

Twin-Flame Crystal

▶ **FACTS:** This type of stone consists of two crystals attached naturally at the sides or joined at the base and forming a V shape. They must be similar but do not have to be identical in size or length, as do the soul mate crystals. This crystal is not the same as the soul mate crystal.

▶ **MAGICAL POWERS:** This double crystal aids in attracting those whose spiritual development matches yours, rather than a romantic attraction. Since this stone connects with past lives, these people may well have known and worked with you before. It will also attract spiritual companions who will be valuable in your growth on all levels.

Veil Crystal

▶ **FACTS:** Sometimes called a wall crystal, this stone will have an inner fracture or inclusion that seems to divide the crystal. This "wall" may appear either solid or gauzy. It is quite possible for a veil crystal to also have rainbows.

▶ **MAGICAL POWERS:** This crystal has two very strong but different abilities. It can be used to create a wall around yourself to keep out undesirable people and their influences, or it can act as a mediator between you and someone else when a wall has been erected and now needs to come down.

Wand Crystal

▶ **FACTS:** Sometimes called a Merlin or laser wand, this crystal is long and thin. The point will be slightly rounded or have only three sides. The wand, or laser wand, crystal is often disappointing in its appearance, as few will be perfectly clear. Frequently, it is dull and dirty looking, deeply etched with grooves, and may have small finger-like crystals at one end.

Natural wand crystals are difficult to find, and expensive when you do find one. However, crystal wands of manmade lead crystal are available at much more reasonable prices. Most of these are excellent and work the same as the natural crystal wands, only on a gentler vibrational level.

Since wand crystals are extremely powerful and their energy concentrated to a fine, cutting point, you should never casually point one at anyone unless you know exactly what you are doing and plan to heal. These crystals are quite capable of slicing or puncturing the aura. However, they can also be used to draw a protective circle about yourself or an object.

▶ **HEALING ENERGIES:** An excellent healing tool, the wand crystal can be used to direct energy right to a diseased area.

▶ **MAGICAL POWERS:** An outstanding shamanic, dream, and soul-rescue stone, the wand crystal focuses and directs energy with pinpoint accuracy. It can be used to destroy any kind of incoming negative vibrations, as well as directing energy during rituals and spellworks for a manifestation. Used during meditation, it will aid in contacting the Higher Self and sending telepathic messages.

Window Crystal 1

▶ **FACTS:** Sometimes called a picture window crystal, this egg-shaped quartz is slightly rounded with a frost-like outer covering. They get their beat-up appearance and rounded shape by being tumbled down riverbeds in Brazil and Alaska. A piece of one end or side will be sliced off, allowing a view of the interior.

▶ **MAGICAL POWERS:** This stone can draw you into meditation merely by gazing into its depths through the sliced window. It is an outstanding shamanic, vision quest, and dream stone. It can also act as a divination tool when scrying.

Window Crystal 2

▶ **FACTS:** The second type of crystal known as a window crystal is a quartz crystal point. The window in this crystal is a large diamond shape at the front. The top point of this diamond will be connected to a line that leads to the apex of the crystal; the side points connect with the angles of the adjoining faces. The bottom point will be connected to a line that runs to the base of the crystal. This window should be large enough to be called a seventh face of the crystal.

▶ **HEALING ENERGIES:** Can be used in a divinatory fashion to diagnose illnesses. To do this, hold the diamond window to the third eye and ask to be shown what is causing the physical or mental problem of the sick person.

▶ **MAGICAL POWERS:** The magical uses of this window crystal are the same as those listed for window crystal 1.

Rhodocrosite

▶ **HARDNESS:** 4

▶ **COLORS:** Shades of pink, strawberry, salmon, or reddish pink, with narrow bands of pale pink or white. Sometimes striped with peach, cream, or milky white.

▶ **SOURCES:** Argentina, Mexico, Namibia, Spain, Romania, Russia, Colorado, and Montana.

▶ **FACTS:** Although gem-quality crystals do occur on occasion, most rhodochrosite is fine-grained, banded rock. It is found in veins with manganese, copper, silver, and lead. The oldest rhodochrosite mines are in Argentina; this Argentinean stone is sometimes called Inca Rose.

▶ **HISTORY AND FOLKLORE:** The name rhodocrosite comes from the Greek *rhodon*, meaning pink.

Before World War II, rhodochrosite was discovered at San Luis in Argentina. The Argentine stone is often called Inca Rose because the Incas left evidence that they worked the same mines earlier. The Incas believed that the blood of their ancient rulers turned into this stone.[50]

Rhodochrosite is also found in deep red crystals, especially at Hotazel, South Africa.

This stone is sometimes associated with the signs of Leo and Scorpio.

To dream of rhodochrosite symbolizes an unresolved emotional issue that is troubling you.

▶ **HEALING ENERGIES:** Heals disorders of the stomach and respiratory system.

▶ **MAGICAL POWERS:** Soothes the nervous system, enhances the immune system, and helps the circulation of blood. Because it is an emotional balancer, it can heal emotional wounds and help resolve emotional traumas. An aid to the memory and intellect, this stone also helps to bring an acceptance of the self and life, and mends tears in the aura. A powerful healer for those attuned to it, this stone can align all the subtle bodies. Helps the wearer to access memories from the present and past lives.

Associated with the lower three chakras, rhodocrosite can be used to clear away unresolved emotional issues, which may have created troublesome blockages. This stone can also help you discover your purpose in life.

Can magnetize, strengthen, then hold the energy field around the wearer or an area. Has a strong effect on intuition and creativity. Enhances the dream state.

MAGICAL USES

When doing a divination of any kind, put a piece of rhodocrosite on each of the four corners of the table, or in a square around the area on which you lay out the cards, throw the runes, or whatever. The stones will help you to access past life information that has a bearing on the present day question being asked. Many times, we look too much to the future, rather than the past, for answers to why things are not going as we want them to.

Rhodonite

▶ **HARDNESS:** 5.5–6.5

▶ **COLORS:** Pink, rose red, or purplish red with thin veins or patches of gray to black.

▶ **SOURCES:** The Ural Mountains in Russia, Sweden, Australia, Brazil,

Mexico, the U.S., Canada, Italy, India, Madagascar, South Africa, Japan, New Zealand, and England.

► **FACTS:** The name comes from the Greek word *rhodos* (rose). This very distinct pink or reddish pink stone most often has black veins of manganese-rich material running through it. The massive rhodonite can be opaque to translucent and is used for carving. The rare, fragile crystals are transparent.

► **HISTORY AND FOLKLORE:** This stone was first used in Russia in the late eighteenth century. Its rose red color, usually with black veins, was fashioned into cabochons, beads, vases, boxes, goblets, and other ornamental objects. One of the major sources of rhodonite is still the Ural Mountains in Russia.

  Some writers connect this stone with the sign of Taurus.

  To dream of rhodonite refers to stress in your life.

► **HEALING ENERGIES:** Helps the nervous system, thyroid, pituitary gland, and the body reflexes. Also strengthens the immune system. Aids the heart.

► **MAGICAL POWERS:** By reducing stress and calming the mind, it can ease physical and emotional traumas. This stone enhances self-esteem, confidence, and the energy levels of both the body and mind. Excellent for all healers or spiritual seekers who must live and/or work within metropolitan areas.

  Pink with brown, yellow, or gray markings: aids in keeping your dignity and temper when under stress.

  Pink or pink with black markings: gives an aura of elegance and grace. By helping to release anxiety, this stone helps one to reach one's maximum potential. Very good for sensitive people who want to be left in peace by those of both the physical and astral planes.

MAGICAL USES

If you find yourself getting interrupted too much, being the recipient of unwanted visitors (physical or astral), or just need some quiet time by yourself, wear or carry rhodonite. Put a piece of this stone on your desk as a psychic barrier. Place it on your coffee table to deter physical visitors, by your bed to deter astral visitors. The astral visitors need not be the really unwelcome kind for you to use this method.

Perhaps the astral teachers and visitors are merely keeping you so busy at night that you are tired in the morning. A piece of rhodonite is a kind of "do not bother" sign to them, saying you need a vacation.

Rose Quartz: see Quartz

Ruby

- ► **HARDNESS:** 9
- ► **COLORS:** Usually true shades of red, but can occur in pinkish red, purplish red, fiery vermilion, or brownish red.
- ► **SOURCES:** Myanmar, Thailand, Afghanistan, Pakistan, Vietnam, India, the U.S., Russia, Australia, and Norway.
- ► **FACTS:** Ruby is a type of gem-quality corundum with its crystals found as six-sided prisms. Pure corundum being colorless, the ruby red color is caused by the presence of chromium. The chromium makes rubies fluoresce under ultraviolet light like hot coals. Ruby was once called the carbuncle, or *carbunculus*, which means "a glowing coal."

  One of the most important ways of distinguishing real rubies from manmade ones is by the inclusions naturally found in these stones. These inclusions include needles of rutile, zircon crystals, and liquid-filled cavities.

  The finest quality rubies, whose color is compared to pigeon's blood, are found in Burma. Rubies from Thailand have small traces of iron which give a slightly brownish tint to the stones, while those from Sri Lanka are more pink than red. The very palest pink rubies are sold under the name of pink sapphire, sapphire being another corundum.

  In 1996, a 9 1/2-pound ruby of over 21,000 carats was found in Myanmar. It is so flawless that the government says it cannot be valued.
- ► **HISTORY AND FOLKLORE:** The gem traders of Bangkok, Thailand, still tell the old legend of how the color of rubies ripens and matures from pure white to red in the ground over thousands of years. Another Burmese legend tells of the great dragon Naga who

laid three magical eggs long ago: the first egg held Pyusawti, king of Burma; the second, the great Chinese emperor; and the third, all the rubies in the world. The favorite gem of Burma, the ruby at one time was said to give invulnerability if inserted in the flesh.

One of the titles of the ancient kings of Burma was "Lord of the Rubies." Whenever the miners found a large, beautiful ruby, the king sent a procession of nobles to the mines, accompanied by a military escort mounted on elephants. The ruby was taken back to the palace where it was received with solemn ceremonies. This respect of the Hindus may have influenced the ruby's importance in Arabic countries; it figures prominently in the Koran.

A Hindu legend says that the ruby was at first colorless like a diamond. When a maharani was stabbed to death by a jealous court attendant, her blood stained her colorless rubies a blood red; all other rubies turned this shade in response.

The Hindus highly prized rubies, which they believed protected their owners from ill fortune. They refused to keep the true, greater rubies with any flawed ones, lest the better rubies lose their virtues. The ruby has many names in Sanskrit, among them *ratnaraj* ("king of precious stones"), *rananayaka* ("leader of precious stones"), and *padmaraga* ("red as the lotus"). They believed this stone gave the wearer total protection from enemies and misfortune, dispelled evil thoughts, reconciled disputes, and cured disease.

The famous Timur Ruby was mined in India and originally owned by the sultans of Delhi. When Tamerlane of Samarkand invaded the city, he took it as part of his loot. This great ruby eventually passed down to Shah Jehan, who built the Taj Mahal. Later it was taken by the Persian Nadir Shah. After the Shah's assassination in 1747, the stone went to Afghanistan, later to be paid to the British as part of war reparations in the mid-1800s. The Timor Ruby is now part of a necklace worn on state occasions by the British queen.

The famous Peacock Throne of Persia (present-day Iran) was encrusted with thousands of gems, among them 108 rubies.

In the Orient and the Far East, the ruby is said to reveal the presence of poison by changing color, guards the wearer from attacks by enemies, and attracts the best of fortunes. The ancient Chaldeans believed this stone was the most powerful gem for protecting from evil and attracting favors.

The ancient Greek philosopher and naturalist Theophrastus and the Roman writer Pliny both wrote about "male" and "female" rubies. The "males" were supposed to be the more brilliant ones. However, Pliny tended to put all red stones into the same class— rubies, garnets, and red spinels—although he appeared to know the difference. The Greeks called ruby *anthrax*, while the Romans knew it as *carbunculus*.

The British of the time of Queen Elizabeth I were quite impressed by the ruby. Sir Jerome Horsey, trusted messenger to the court of Ivan the Terrible in Russia, reported that Ivan considered the ruby able to improve memory, cleanse the blood, and help the heart.

From the 1300s to the 1600s, physicians strongly believed in the power of the ruby to keep one's health—mental and physical— good. The practice of touching the ruby to the four corners of one's land to protect from lightning, tempests, and poor harvests was also practiced during this time. Ruby was considered so important that in 1560 it cost eight times as much as diamond.

Madame de Pompadour, mistress of the French king Louis XV, had a large ruby cut in the shape of a pig, which she wore for good luck. This ruby is now in the Louvre Museum.

For centuries the ruby has been said to banish sadness, prevent nightmares, and protect the wearer from plagues. It was also believed to stop hemorrhages and cure inflammations. Physicians in the Middle East frequently prescribed finely ground ruby in fruit juice for apprehension, diseased livers, and eye problems. The ruby was also said to darken when danger was near.

Like the garnet, the ruby is considered a warrior's stone. Warriors of many Asian and Malaysian countries believed that a fine ruby made a man invulnerable to all weapons made of steel. To secure this invincibility, however, the ruby had to be inserted between the skin and the flesh.

Star rubies—those whose inclusions form a star pattern—are considered to be of very great value all over the Orient. Legend says the star is formed by three benign spirits, who have been imprisoned inside the stone for some minor infraction. The translation of the names of these spirits are Faith, Hope, and Destiny. These same spirits are said to live within star sapphires. Anyone who possessed a star ruby is assured that his or her fortune will change for the better.

Aries, Leo, Scorpio, and Cancer have been associated with the ruby. This stone is said to be ruled by Mars.

To dream of a ruby means great love. It can also symbolize unexpected guests.

▶ **HEALING ENERGIES:** A vitalizer of the whole body, mind, and circulatory system, this stone can activate sluggish conditions on both the physical and spiritual levels. Cleans the chakras from the heart downward.

▶ **MAGICAL POWERS:** Working with this stone can remove all sense of limitation. Strengthens courage, selfless work, spiritual endeavors, joy, and leadership qualities. Helps to reduce resentment when you have to care for others.

The ruby can produce a strong sense and means of power within a person; this power should be handled responsibly or it can turn into anger and possessive thoughts. Aids in intuitive thinking.

Although physically the ruby represents passionate love, in esoteric terms it symbolizes spiritual love reached through transformation. It signifies wisdom that is raised to the higher vibration of divine wisdom. A protective and stabilizing stone, the ruby can help one deal with grief on all levels, and it also attracts friends.

MAGICAL USES

Many people like to wear the ruby around the Winter Solstice, never realizing that, although the red color goes with the season, they also enjoy wearing the stone for its subconscious energy of strength, joy, and spirituality. Of course, these energies are valuable whenever you wear a ruby, so put one on when you have to go for a job interview, seek the advice of an attorney, or during any time when you want to feel and appear in control and happy with yourself. Wear the ruby where the other person with whom you are talking will see it: earrings or necklace is best. Unless you plan to wave a ring before the person's face all the time, the ruby will not be in constant view.

As a love stone, ruby represents physical passion as the rose quartz represents the sweeter true-love aspect. The sale of rubies goes up around Valentine's Day when spouses and lovers want to present their mate with a gift.

Bypass jewelry stores when seeking rubies and other precious stones, unless you just particularly want a flashy piece of jewelry. Too many times, these stores will advertise precious gems as authentic when they are actually synthetic. Synthetic is just as useful to the magician, but why pay big money because of false advertising? Unset, faceted, or tumbled gemstones are much cheaper from smaller rock dealers or individual jewelry makers.

Be careful about using the ruby in any love spells. The only way you can temper its highly sexual energy is to pair a single ruby with several pieces of rose quartz. Hopefully, you will want to attract someone who will stay in your life as a lover, not a one-night stand.

Sapphire

- ▶ **HARDNESS:** 9
- ▶ **COLORS:** Variations of blue, from cornflower to deep midnight blue, which is almost black. Other colors are white, green, violet, yellow, brown, orange, and pink.
- ▶ **SOURCES:** Myanmar, Sri Lanka, India, Thailand, Australia, Nigeria, Montana, Cambodia, Brazil, Kenya, Colombia, Tanzania, and Malawi.
- ▶ **FACTS:** The sapphire is a corundum like the ruby. Ruby and sapphire are the second hardest stones in the world, next to diamonds. The name sapphire probably came from the Greek word *sapphiros* ("beloved of Saturn"[51]) or *sapheiros*, which came from a Sanskrit word. The Persians knew this stone as *saffir* and the Arabs as *safir*. The Latin word *sapphirus* used by Pliny the Elder also referred to lapis lazuli.

In 1880, a small deposit of the best quality sapphires ever seen was discovered in Kashmir; unfortunately, these were mined out long ago. Now the best of the dark royal blue color is marketed under the name of *Kanchanaburi* (from the mines where it is found), but these mines are also fast being depleted. Stones of several carats are almost as valuable as diamonds and rubies. Sapphires of cornflower blue are considered to be the finest hue and the most valuable.

Although the sapphire is commonly thought of as a beautiful, rich blue stone, it comes in a variety of colors. In fact, every corundum not red is a sapphire. The only other corundum to have its separate name is the very rare and expensive *padparadscha*, Sinhalese for "lotus blossom." This gemstone is pinkish orange and is only found in Sri Lanka.

Yellow sapphires range from pale shades to brownish yellow. Most of it is mined in Sri Lanka, with only a small amount coming from Australia and Burma. Once called the Oriental topaz, yellow sapphire can be difficult to distinguish from yellow chrysoberyl.

The greens come mainly from Australia, but are also found in Montana and Thailand. Once called the Oriental emerald, green sapphires range from bright green to bluish green and even into yellowish green. Although their value is low, they are scarce.

Pink sapphire can range from very delicate shades to a pink with a slight violet tinge; although this color is less valuable than the blue, it is more highly prized. Pinks found in Burma are rare.

Sapphires ranging from violet to violet blue, violet red, and violet pink were once called Oriental amethyst. Most stones of these colors come from Sri Lanka; however, they are also found in Thailand and Burma.

Colorless sapphire can be perfectly without color, with a slight yellow tint, or have fine, crossed needles of rutile. At one time it was known as leucosapphire (from the Greek word *leykos*, meaning "white"). Found in only one place now, Sri Lanka, white sapphire is connected with Venus and often substituted for the diamond as April's birthstone.

The most rare and expensive of all sapphires is the star sapphire. This sapphire shows *asterism*, or a six-rayed star, when included rutile needles are parallel to the three crystal axes and the stone is cut *en cabochon.*

▶ **HISTORY AND FOLKLORE:** For many centuries, all blue stones were called sapphires, so it is very difficult to determine what stone was actually meant in some historical writings. However, the history of the use of sapphire can accurately be traced back to the Etruscan in the seventh century B.C.E.

Held in great reverence by eastern religions, the sapphire is called the "Stone of Stones" by the Buddhists, who say this stone will give peace of mind, happiness, and spiritual enlightenment. The Hindus believe that sapphire is one of the mystical gems, with blue sapphire granting good health, wealth, happiness, and the blessings of the deities. The Greeks considered the sapphire a stone of Apollo and believed it could kill spiders.

Ancient Persian legend says that sapphires came into existence from the last drops of the elixir of immortality, the *amrita.* This substance was also known as the life-giving milk of the Goddess.[52]

The Hebrews believe that a sapphire was the seal-stone in King Solomon's ring. During the Middle Ages in Europe, the sapphire was believed to preserve chastity, uncover fraud and treachery, protect from black magic, and repel the plague. In France, during the thirteenth century, this stone was carried to ward off poverty.

In the twelfth century C.E., Christian clergy adopted sapphire for ecclesiastical rings with such fervor that Pope Innocent III finally issued a decree that every bishop should wear a gold ring with a sapphire set in it. However, many of the surviving rings have turned out to be only blue paste or opaque glass.[53]

The St. Edward's Sapphire, now set in the cross-straps of the British Imperial State Crown, has a fanciful legend behind it. King Edward the Confessor is supposed to have given his sapphire ring to a beggar. Years later the ring was returned to the king with the message, "I will meet you in paradise." The king died shortly afterwards, and the ring was buried with him. After 200 years, Edward's coffin was opened, the ring taken out and put on display in Westminster Abbey. The touch of this sapphire was supposed to cure paralysis, epilepsy, and failing sight.

Powdered sapphire mixed with milk was applied to boils and other skin eruptions during the Middle Ages. The brilliant blue color was also used as an antidote to poisons and poisonous bites. Sapphire was used by physicians to treat fevers, agues, skin disorders, stomach ulcers, plague, and eye diseases. In the seventeenth century, a large sapphire was given to the Church of St. Paul's in London for this healing purpose.

Sapphire was also known in the Middle East as a stone of love. The sorcerers of the court of Haroun el Raschid, Emperor of the East, made a special love talisman for the Emperor Charlemagne (800–814 C.E.) to give his wife. This talisman had one oval sapphire and one square sapphire set into a cross supposedly of the wood from the true cross. The idea behind this talisman may have originated in the Eastern belief that all star sapphires are inhabited by three good spirits who bring good fortune, faith, and hope.

However, other cultures called star sapphires the Stones of Destiny; their three crossing rays were said to invoke the Triple Fate Goddess. Ancient traditions say that the star sapphire was a bearer of good fortune in the most complete sense. Eastern tradition ascribed the same meaning to starred rubies.

Sir Richard Burton, who traveled all over the Middle East, has a large star sapphire, or asteria, that he believed was his talisman of good luck. The people of the area thought that just looking at a star sapphire was lucky, so Burton always brought out his stone and was given good horses and prompt attention in return.

The largest star sapphire on record was the Star of India, which weighed in at 543 carats. These Asteria, or Star Stones, were thought to be extra powerful for bringing good fortune and love and averting evil sorcery.

In ancient Greece, all supplicants to the Oracle of the god Apollo were required to wear a blue sapphire. In the Greek legend of Prometheus, who stole fire from heaven for humans, this Titan was said to have worn a sapphire ring.

It was believed in ancient times that all sorcerers and witches used sapphires to fix enchantments and spells and to understand divinations. During the Middle Ages, sorcerers and magicians often controlled the people in their village or town by saying that the blue sapphire would change to a violet color in the presence of infidelity. It was also said that this stone could point out fraud, treachery, and enchantments, as well as protect from envy and revenge by enemies. If worn by a psychic person, this stone is said to warn of hidden dangers.

The sapphire is associated with the signs of Virgo, Libra, and Sagittarius.

To dream of sapphire means protection from danger.

▶ **HEALING ENERGIES:** By enhancing the activity of the pituitary gland, it helps the entire glandular system. Wear over the heart to reduce fever. Heals the mind and spirit. Helpful for backaches and skin problems; also said to improve the hair and nails. There are some claims that the sapphire helps to heal cancer.

▶ **MAGICAL POWERS:** Excellent for meditation as it breaks up confusion. Aligns the body, mind, and spirit, as well as stimulating the psychic abilities and inspiration. Can help in communication with the Higher Self and spirit guides. Intensifies spellworking, creative expression, and cosmic awareness. Helps in transforming the spiritual life and ambitions. Excellent for learning the higher mysteries. Breaks up old blockages and seals the aura. Will focus energy without the conscious effort of the wearer.

A very old tradition says that a sapphire of any color will dissolve poverty and replace it with prosperity.

According to the Buddhist tradition, a sapphire has special powers that will induce a trance. This stone will also aid with astral projection, channeling, and the development of psychic powers.

Dark blue: ruled by Jupiter, this stone intensifies the creativity and all its potentials; provides grounding for creative people and helps them to follow through on projects. Creates a sense of loyalty in relationships. Aids in developing intuition and clairvoyance. Breaks through illusions to reveal the truth. A Saturn stone, this color of sapphire will dissolve negatives in the conscious and subconscious, and replace them with more illumination.

Green: a good-luck stone, it creates a prosperous attitude and atmosphere.

Light blue: leads one to inspirational thoughts. Encourages positive thoughts about life and what one can accomplish.

Lilac (rare): removes blocks to creativity and progress in life.

Padparadscha (orange): helps with perspective and the gaining of knowledge; excellent for careers in such fields as libraries, writing, and teaching. Strengthens mental wellness and brings happiness; a good healer of the emotions. A good-luck stone in that it attracts wealth and honor, and protects against untimely death.

Pink: relaxes those who feel they always have to be in control.

Star: ruled by Saturn, this form of sapphire projects the message that one wants privacy and will not tolerate interference in one's life. It guards against evil sorcery, often long after it is no longer owned. It also makes Saturn cycles and aspects easier.

White: encourages one to be good to oneself and not so critical and demanding.

Yellow: helps to learn and retain information; aids in the access of knowledge.

MAGICAL USES

Any color of sapphire is so beneficial, I recommend that every person should wear one for the positive vibrations alone. If you are into magical and spiritual seeking, the sapphire is a must, whether you wear the stone or merely use it for rituals. This gem is a great help to anyone who has an afflicted Saturn in her/his natal chart, or is experiencing problems with Saturn transits.

Sard

▶ **HARDNESS:** 7
▶ **COLOR:** Reddish brown; similar to agate.
▶ **SOURCE:** Found worldwide.
▶ **FACTS:** A type of chalcedony, which is a microcrystalline quartz. The reddish brown form of chalcedony that was called sard in ancient history we now know as carnelian.
▶ **HISTORY AND FOLKLORE:** The Greeks called this stone *sarx*

("flesh"), from its color. Through the time of Swedenborg, sard was commonly known as the "sardine stone." Pliny said it got this name from its place of origin in Asia Minor—Sardis.

The Etruscans made beads, scarabs, charms, and ornaments out of sard. Ornaments of this stone have also been found in the ruins of Mycenae (1450–1100 B.C.E.) and Assyria (1400–600 B.C.E.), as well as in later Roman territory.

Sard is connected with Mars and the sign of Aries.

To dream of this stone means a possible change of residence.

▶ **HEALING ENERGIES:** Aids in digestion. Ruled by Mars, at one time this stone was used to heal any wound made by iron.

▶ **MAGICAL POWERS:** Creates a feeling of having roots, family/friend ties; makes one more comfortable within whatever is called home.

Said to be a powerful protector against spells and evil sorcery.

MAGICAL USES

Sard can be used as part of any ritual or spell where you are working magic to get a new, or at least a different, place of residence. If you have to move to another town or state, do a candle ritual with sard on the altar to help you find a suitable home in which to live.

Carry a sard ornament on your key chain or in your purse to deflect negative thoughts or deliberately sent ill-wishing. Place a piece prominently in your home to do the same work.

Sardonyx

▶ **HARDNESS:** 7

▶ **COLORS:** Straight white bands of onyx and brownish red of sard.

▶ **SOURCE:** Worldwide.

▶ **FACTS:** A variety of chalcedony, which is a crystalline quartz. Sardonyx, also known as sardian onyx, is a blend of sard and onyx. Ancient writers considered the only valuable sardonyx was of the colors black, red, and white—the three ancient colors of the Triple Goddess.

▶ **HISTORY AND FOLKLORE:** Sardonyx has been in use for thousands of years. Since it is composed of different colored layers, it has been used to carve seals and cameos. The Romans liked to carve this stone with the image of Mars or Hercules, believing it made the wearer fearless and full of courage.

In Classical times, sardonyx was worn by lawyers, as it was believed to make them more eloquent.

Many ancient cultures credited sardonyx with ensuring a happy marriage, success in legal matters, attracting friends, relieving pain, and protecting from infections and poisonous bites or stings.

Sardonyx is often associated with Virgo.

To dream of sardonyx signifies the love of many friends.

▶ **HEALING ENERGIES:** Unknown.

▶ **MAGICAL POWERS:** Encourages the wearer to be more adventurous and willing to take on challenges in life. Gives self-control, friends, success in business matters that touch upon the law, and good fortune.

A defensive stone, sardonyx is said to dispel sorrow.

MAGICAL USES

Sardonyx can be used in many of the same ways that sard is used. Carry as a good luck stone that will shield and deflect negatives.

Scapolite

▶ **HARDNESS:** 6

▶ **COLORS:** Ranges in color from pink, purple, blue, yellow, and gray to colorless.

▶ **SOURCES:** Brazil, Myanmar, Canada, Kenya, and Madagascar.

▶ **FACTS:** This stone is found in both crystals and the massive form. The crystals are found in stick-like prisms, which accounts for this stone's Greek-based name. The crystals can be cut either *en cabochon* or faceted. The pink and purple cabochons frequently show a cat's-eye effect from their dark mineral inclusions. Scapolite can be easily misidentified as chrysoberyl or golden beryl.

When exposed to X rays or radium, yellow scapolite turns a vivid amethyst purple. However, this induced color always fades, while the naturally purple stone will not.

Scapolite is also called wernerite, after the German geologist A. G. Werner (1750–1817).

▶ **HISTORY AND FOLKLORE:** The name scapolite comes from the Greek words *scapos*, or "rod", and *lithos*, or "stone."

Scapolite is often associated with Uranus and Neptune, as well as the signs of Gemini, Scorpio, and Pisces.

To dream of this stone means you may be changing jobs or careers. It can also refer to your juggling more than one occupation and/or outside activity.

▶ **HEALING ENERGIES:** Unknown.

▶ **MAGICAL POWERS:** This stone is helpful to actors and other people who are required to present more than one persona to the public.

Use in rituals to create very different changes in your life or career.

MAGICAL USES

Scapolite is useful for sending out specific energy: energy for radical changes. Draw upon its power in rituals and spellworkings only if you desire your life to change dramatically. This stone does not bother with minor changes or even degrees of change from the status you already have, but will alter your present reality into a totally different state of existence. For this reason you should be very specific about what you want.

Selenite

▶ **HARDNESS:** 2
▶ **COLORS:** Transparent to opaque; white, gray, other colors.
▶ **SOURCE:** Worldwide.
▶ **FACTS:** A clear variety of gypsum, selenite crystals often form as seawater evaporates. As they become heavier, these crystals sink to the

seabed. Selenite crystals have a glassy luster, are easily chipped, and are damaged if exposed to water.

Some selenite crystals form into long, smooth natural wands, which can be quite spectacular. The Cave of Swords in Mexico has selenite specimens that are up to five feet tall.

▶ **HISTORY AND FOLKLORE:** Although the name selenite means moonstone, it has no connection with the other more beautiful and durable moonstones listed in this book. Its silvery quality does remind one of moonlight, however. Selene was the Greek goddess of the Moon.

Selenite is associated with the Moon and the sign of Cancer.

To dream of this stone means a pleasant period where you and your home will be the center of positive social interactions.

▶ **HEALING ENERGIES:** Although this stone helps the body to assimilate needed vitamins and minerals, do not ingest it. The stone should be laid on the body or run over the aura to gain the effect.

▶ **MAGICAL POWERS:** Can be used to cleanse and recharge other stones. Enhances mental clarity and efficiency.

MAGICAL USES

Never cleanse selenite in water, as it will be permanently damaged. Selenite is most useful in the cleansing and charging of other gemstones. Using either a selenite spear or a round selenite mushroom formation, set the stone or stones on the selenite and leave for about an hour. You can also use a selenite spear in another fashion for cleansing. Put a gemstone near the spear's pointed end and leave it for a time.[54]

Serpentine

▶ **HARDNESS:** 2–3
▶ **COLORS:** Shades of green and blue-green.
▶ **SOURCES:** Bowenite is mined in New Zealand, China, Afghanistan, South Africa, and the U.S. Williamsite is found in Italy, England, and China.
▶ **FACTS:** Serpentine is actually a group of primarily green minerals. It

grows in masses of very small intergrown crystals rather than in individual crystals of any size. There are two main types of serpentine: bowenite (translucent green or blue-green) and williamsite (translucent green, veined with inclusions). Williamsite is the rare variety of this stone. Both bowenite and williamsite are engraved, carved, or polished.

▶ **HISTORY AND FOLKLORE:** Another name for this stone is snake-stone, because the pattern of its colors often resembles a snake's scales and patterning.

Serpentine is associated with the sign of Scorpio.

To dream of this stone symbolizes treachery from someone.

▶ **HEALING ENERGIES:** Unknown.

▶ **MAGICAL POWERS:** Has much the same effects as jade. Increases wisdom and self-restraint. Should be worn on a cord rather than a chain.

A stone of Scorpio, serpentine is said to protect against venomous bites of all kinds.

MAGICAL USES

Carved serpentine is quite lovely and makes an interesting and pretty piece of jewelry. Use it in rituals according to the corresponding color of jade; the uses are almost identical.

Shell

▶ **HARDNESS:** 3

▶ **COLORS:** Many colors.

▶ **SOURCES:** In seas and oceans around the world.

▶ **FACTS:** Mother-of-pearl and Paua shell is simply the dark blue and pearly silver lining of an abalone shell. The abalone basically has a large flattened shell with small holes that the creature uses to breathe. It is distributed worldwide, with the larger species living in temperate waters.

Cowrie shells are small elliptical shells with a convex base and sometimes a little humped back. They range in size from very tiny up to 3 1/2 to 4 inches in length. They are found in the Caribbean and Indo-Pacific oceans, where they live on coral reefs and around rocks. The aperture on the base, or under side, of the cowrie is ridged with short teeth-like projections; this is where the mantle of the creature protrudes from the shell. The golden cowry, one of the larger of the species, is highly prized.

The scallop is the best known of all the bivalve creatures. Scallop shells have a wide fan-shape with two "ears" at the pointed base of the shell. There are a great many species of scallop. The great scallop's shell was featured in Botticelli's painting of Venus; this shell can vary in color from white to brown. The Asian Moon scallop is found in the Indo-Pacific Ocean, and the shell of one species is a brilliant white. Perhaps the most distinctive scallop is called the lion's paw, a scallop found in Caribbean waters. The lion's paw has a thick, heavy shell that is twice as wide as it is long. It is a purplish brown on the inside of the shell, while the outside is a variety of red, orange, and yellow.

There are hundreds of types of shells, from the long, pointed auger shells to the twisting cones, to the varieties of clam, to the tritons, and many others. The most fascinating to me are the conches and the trumpets, which can reach up to 30 inches in length.

▶ **HISTORY AND FOLKLORE:** Shells, particularly the cowrie shell, have been used as decorations, amulets, and religious objects as far back as 20,000 B.C.E. The cowrie was known to the Romans as *matriculus* ("the little womb"); they also called it *porcella*, which means both vulva and little sow.[55] Throughout the Mediterranean civilizations, the Middle East, and the Pacific, the little cowrie shell was used both as a Goddess symbol and to work magic for healing, fertility, rebirth, and good luck. The magical use of this shell continued well into the Christian era.

The scallop shell also has a long history of religious significance. These shells have been found in goddess shrines throughout the Mediterranean area, Europe, and into the British Isles. The scallop shell was one symbol of the Celtic goddess Brigit, who is another form of Aphrodite.[56] This shell's use as a yoni symbol of the

Goddess can be traced from the English word *scallop* back to the Norse word *skalpr* ("a sheath" or "vulva").[57]

All shells are associated with the element of Water.

To dream of shells symbolized a new beginning or birth coming.

▶ **HEALING ENERGIES:** Mother-of-pearl and abalone: very healing to the body and especially to the first three chakras.

Abalone: calming to high-strung people.

Paua: heals the body of stress-related diseases.

▶ **MAGICAL POWERS:** All shells offer a connection with the Goddess and Water deities. They are also valuable when working through emotional situations, past or present.

Auger: good for rituals to pierce through walls that are keeping you from progressing.

Clams: draws in prosperity and money.

Conch and trumpet: excellent for connecting with Water deities. Meditating with them, as with other types of shells, can draw you into the astral spiral path that can lead to past lives.

Cowrie: helps with fertility and fertile ideas.

Paua: very useful when facing times of heavy karma or soul transformations.

MAGICAL USES

An abalone shell makes a beautiful ritual accessory. It can be filled with a layer of sand and used as an incense burner, or used as a vessel to hold small items. A scallop shell can be used in the same way.

If you are ever fortunate enough to get a large conch or trumpet shell, it can be used as a prime connection with Water deities. If you do not mind altering its natural shape, you can get a knowledgeable person to trim one end so you can blow through it. This makes a mournful, eerie sound that would certainly get the attention of all at a gathering when you signal in this way for the ceremonies to begin.

Decorating any altar with a collection of shells, whatever their size, is an appropriate way to honor the Goddess. Sometimes you can find necklaces made of little pieces of tumbled and smoothed shell; these are quite lovely and are very nice to wear during rituals.

Smoky Quartz: see Quartz

Sodalite

▶ **HARDNESS:** 5.5

▶ **COLORS:** All shades of blue.

▶ **SOURCES:** Brazil, Canada, India, Namibia, and the U.S. The rare, small twelve-sided crystals are found in the lava beds of the Vesuvius volcano.

▶ **FACTS:** Sodalite is usually found in the massive form, rather than crystals. Its name is derived from its sodium content. This stone is frequently found with lapis lazuli, but contains little or no golden pyrite specks in it as lapis does. It may, however, contain patches or streaks of white calcite. Although some people think that sodalite resembles lapis in some ways, it is entirely different in chemical composition and has more of a navy blue coloring.

The biggest commercial source of sodalite is in Bancroft, Canada. It was found while Princess Margaret was visiting the area, and is sometimes known as Princess Blue.

▶ **HISTORY AND FOLKLORE:** There are no records to show whether this stone was recognized by ancient peoples.

Sodalite can be connected with the sign of Sagittarius.

To dream of this stone means a conflict will soon be ended.

▶ **HEALING ENERGIES:** By balancing the endocrine system, it strengthens the metabolism. Reduces stress and helps to prolong physical endurance. Helpful in lowering both blood pressure and fevers.

▶ **MAGICAL POWERS:** Although sodalite's energies and powers resemble those of lapis lazuli, these are on a milder level. However, its powers can be amplified if you use it with other blue gemstones. This stone can balance male and female polarities as well as calming and clearing the mind. Its slightly sedative nature grounds and cuts through illusion. By creating an inner harmony, sodalite can stop or ease any conflicts between the conscious and subconscious minds; it does this by helping you to face reality, release the past, and set positive goals for the future. Sodalite also helps to clear out old mental patterns from the subconscious.

It can strongly affect your attitudes concerning yourself. Sodalite is one of the stones that will open the third eye and bring in inner psychic sight and intuitive knowledge.

Enhances communication abilities and creativity as well as enhancing sensuality. It can also balance and activate the second chakra.

MAGICAL USES

Sodalite is excellent for psychic development and meditation, particularly if used with lapis lazuli and/or clear quartz crystal. Rather than blasting open the inner doorway to the psychic, this stone gently eases it open. This makes acceptance of and working with the new and different abilities much easier than if they came on too suddenly.

Worn in jewelry, sodalite forms a reliable connection with your intuition, thus giving you a gentle flow of information that can save you lots of time and trouble.

Sphalerite

▶ **HARDNESS:** 3.5–4

▶ **COLORS:** Usually very dark brown to black, but occasionally will be transparent, yellowish brown, or green. On rare occasions, this stone will be found in colorless, yellow, or pink.

▶ **SOURCES:** Spain and Mexico.

▶ **FACTS:** Sphalerite crystals are generally found with other minerals, such as galena, quartz, pyrite, and calcite. It is very similar to galena and is an important ore of zinc. Because it is so soft and has perfect cleavage, it is primarily cut and faceted only for museums and collectors and not worn in jewelry. A few suitable stones for cutting have been found, however. When faceted, sphalerite does have a high fire with rainbow colors.

This stone's name comes from the Greek word *sphaleros* ("deceiver"). This is because of its metallic luster and heavy weight, which in some ways resembles iron. Its alternate name, blende, comes from the German word *blendet und betrugt*, which also means deceiver. No useful purpose for sphalerite was found until after 1734, when it was discovered to be the principal source of zinc.

Black sphalerite has a separate name—marmatite—after Marmato, Italy, the locality in which it is found.[58]

▶ **HISTORY AND FOLKLORE:** None known.

Sphalerite can be associated with Neptune, Pluto, and the sign of Pisces.

To dream of this stone signifies a deep need to build up the spiritual side of your life.

▶ **HEALING ENERGIES:** Unknown.

▶ **MAGICAL POWERS:** Use for spiritual awareness and transcending the ego. Moves the wearer beyond the influence of petty problems.

MAGICAL USES

Sphalerite is almost entirely a stone best used for spiritual work rather than mundane goals. It can help, through meditation, spell-working, and ritual, to lift your aspirations to a higher level and aid you in setting your sights on developing the spiritual side of your life. Its vibrations can be so etheric that it is best used no more than once a week. Too frequent use may leave you feeling spacey and a little out of touch with the physical and mundane side of your existence.

Spinel

▶ **HARDNESS:** 8
▶ **COLOR:** Variety of colors.
▶ **SOURCE:** Sri Lanka, Thailand, Burma, and Afghanistan.
▶ **FACTS:** A member of the same mineral group as lodestone, red spinel varies from an intense ruby red to brick red to almost orange and soft pink. It was also known as the carbuncle, along with the ruby and other intensely red stones. The Black Prince's Ruby in the English crown turned out to be a red spinel. Both red and pink spinels are found in Burma, Afghanistan, Sri Lanka, and Thailand.

The blue spinel is mostly found in Sri Lanka and, on rare occasions, in Burma. It ranges in color from bright blue to light violet blue with a sooty gray undertone. Dark green spinel is also called Ceylonite.

The spinel has no electrical properties when subjected to heat, as do the ruby and garnet.

▶ **HISTORY AND FOLKLORE:** The name spinel comes from *spina* ("thorn"), a Latin word that refers to the triangular shape of the crystal faces; another source of the name may be the Greek word *spinos* or *spinter* ("spark"). The Arabic word *balakhsh* may be the origin of the word balas, another name by which this stone was once known. It was called the balas ruby, after its source in the Balascia region of Afghanistan. A Persian tradition says the balas rubies were discovered after an earthquake destroyed a mountain. In India, this stone was called *Lal Rumani* ("pomegranate ruby").

Camillus Leonardus in 1502 wrote that the spinel, as well as the ruby, was useful in treating liver diseases; he also recorded that this stone had the added benefit of protecting the owner and his home from thunderstorms.

One of the biggest hoaxes in history was the Black Prince's Ruby, a stone in the British crown that was thought for centuries to be a ruby.[59] In the 1940s it was discovered that the "ruby" was actually a large red spinel, worth only about twenty dollars.

Spinel is connected with Pluto and Mars and the sign of Aries.

To dream of this stone is a warning to take care in signing any contracts or papers; there may be hidden conditions not to your favor.

▶ **HEALING ENERGIES:** A high-energy stone that can heal physical energy blockages.

▶ **MAGICAL POWERS:** A good-luck stone for the medical profession, secretaries, writers, and business people. Clarifies thoughts and creative ideas. Attracts needed help.

Place at each of the four corners of a house or building to protect against disasters and storms.

Black: helps one be in charge of situations and handle other people in a correct manner.

Blue or gray: enhances discrimination, especially about who are friends and what situations one becomes involved in; good for spiritual communication.

Dark green: increases communication skills; also increases money.

Light green: wear when you feel afraid.

Peach: builds self-esteem and softens criticism toward others or oneself.

Pink: good for couples in relationships as it fosters love.

Red: excellent for vitality, confidence, and leadership.

Violet: use to avoid being victimized; helps communication between generations.

Yellow: good for those with low self-esteem as it fosters belief in one's abilities.

MAGICAL USES

Wear or carry violet spinel when you have to deal with dictatorial older family members, particularly if they have manipulated you in the past. If you have a bad habit of being unnecessarily critical of others, and are vocal about it, wear peach spinel to calm down your need to ridicule. Peach is also good if you are too critical of yourself. This stone in dark green is excellent for attracting money; wear it, or use it in spellworkings as a focal point for the energy. If you already have lots of energy and are fairly aggressive in leadership, do not wear red spinel—it can make you overbearing.

Staurolite

▶ **HARDNESS:** 7

▶ **COLORS:** Reddish brown to brown and black, with tinges of red or orange.

▶ **SOURCES:** Switzerland, Germany, Russia, Brazil, France, Scotland, and the U.S. Very fine staurolite crystals are found in Patrick County, Virginia.

▶ **FACTS:** Sometimes called the Cross Stone, *lapis crucifer* ("stone cross"), Faery Stone or Faery Cross, staurolite is usually an opaque, cross-shaped stone. These twinned crystals can cross at 60-degree (an X) or 90-degree (a Greek cross) angles. Well-formed natural staurolite crosses are rare. Cross stones have been used as amulets and in religious jewelry for centuries.

When broken or sliced, this stone displays a cross pattern of alternating light and dark colors. See Andalusite.

One type of staurolite containing blue cobalt is found in Africa; called lusakite, it is found in Lusaka, Zambia. An even rarer zinc-containing staurolite will change from yellowish green in daylight to reddish brown in artificial light.[60]

▶ **HISTORY AND FOLKLORE:** The name staurolite comes from the Greek word for cross. A paper published in Stockholm in 1758 says that sometimes this stone was known as *Baseler Taufstein* and was used as an amulet at baptisms. Known in Italy as *piedra della croce*, the cross stone is still carried in little bags around the neck or in the pocket as protection against sicknesses caused by dark sorcery. In early Britain, sailors carried the cross stone as protection against disaster at sea. In Brittany, tradition says the staurolites drop from the skies; they are worn as powerful charms.

Shamans in various cultures around the world have long carried staurolite in their medicine bags.

Staurolite is connected with the Earth element.

To dream of staurolite symbolizes a need for balance in your life.

▶ **HEALING ENERGIES:** Good for when you do not feel well but cannot pinpoint the cause.

▶ **MAGICAL POWERS:** Helps to remember past lives, particularly the most distant ones. Easily programmed to carry any vibrations you want, it is a stone of good fortune. Use in rituals to balance the four elements.

MAGICAL USES

Staurolite makes an excellent good-luck and protection amulet to wear or carry. Used in rituals and spellworking, this stone will attract the attention and aid of Nature spirits and other such beings.

Steatite

▶ **HARDNESS:** 1

▶ **COLOR:** Gray-green.

▶ **SOURCE:** In the U.S., large deposits are found in Virginia and the Appalachian Mountain chain from New England to Georgia. Other sources are Manchuria, France, Italy, Canada, India, Norway, and Spain.

▶ **FACTS:** Also known as soapstone, steatite has a greasy luster caused by the abundance of talc in its chemical composition. Because it is resistant to high temperatures and acids, it is often used for laboratory tables, sinks, laundry tubs, and electric panel boards. It is also used by sculptors for carving.

▶ **HISTORY AND FOLKLORE:** None known, except that ancient cultures used the stone for carving.

Steatite can be associated with Aries, Gemini, and Libra.

If you dream of soapstone, or steatite, it means you need to take a firmer stand regarding the way people use and treat you.

▶ **HEALING ENERGIES:** Unknown.

▶ **MAGICAL POWERS:** Same effects as jade.

MAGICAL USES

Use as a substitute for jade.

Sugilite

▶ **COLORS:** Royal, magenta purple.

▶ **SOURCES:** Japan, India, and Africa.

▶ **FACTS:** Also called Royal Lavulite, this stone was first discovered in Japan in 1944; it was named after the Japanese petrologist Kenichi Sugi. Later, other deposits were found in India and Africa. The African sugilite, from the Wessels mine in the Kalahari Desert, is known as wesselsite.

Sugilite was first introduced to Americans at the Tucson Mineral Show in 1981, under the name Royal Lavulite. The next year a California company marketed this stone under the name Royal Azel.

An expensive stone, even small pieces of sugilite bring high prices.

► **HISTORY AND FOLKLORE:** None known.

Sugilite can be connected with Aquarius and Libra.

To dream of sugilite suggests that your spiritual teachers and guides are trying to contact you.

► **HEALING ENERGIES:** Balances and heals all chakras and bodily areas connected with them. Aids in revealing the stresses that caused an illness.

► **MAGICAL POWERS:** Opens the mind and subconscious to higher influences. A very powerful channeling stone, it aids in using psychic powers. Helps in understanding negative circumstances by showing what is out of balance. Excellent for meditation exercises to bring the mind and spirit back into attunement. A spiritual stone, sugilite can help in lifting the thoughts into higher realms of consciousness.

MAGICAL USES

The vibrational energies of sugilite are best used by wearing small stones in jewelry. This gives a constant flow of the stone's magical qualities directly into your aura. However, if you are not greatly interested in spiritual goals and studies, I suggest you bypass this stone and work with others.

Sunstone

► **HARDNESS:** 6–6.5
► **COLORS:** (Manmade) coppery-like or tangerine color with metallic glitter. (Natural) a translucent red.
► **SOURCES:** Norway, the U.S., India, Russia, and Canada.
► **FACTS:** True sunstone is a species of plagioclase feldspar and is

sometimes called aventurine feldspar. It has tiny inclusions of hematite, which produce reflections of red, orange, or green glitter. In some ways, the natural sunstone resembles an orange opal. It is usually carved *en cabochon*. There are also whitish, brown, and greenish sunstones, all with flecks of color. At the end of the eighteenth century, this natural stone was discovered on an island in the White Sea. Later, in both North America and at Lake Baikal in Russia, sunstones with a gold luster were found.

Two deposits of sunstone were found in Russia in the late eighteenth and nineteenth centuries; its use became very popular in Russian jewelry. In 1850 another deposit was discovered in Norway.

Manmade sunstone is called Oregon goldstone.

▶ **HISTORY AND FOLKLORE:** Although we know from hints in ancient writings that sunstone from India was used in magic, we do not know the details.

This stone is associated with the Sun and the sign of Leo.

To dream of sunstone symbolizes approaching success.

▶ **HEALING ENERGIES:** Heals on a cellular level; energizes. Place in a bag of herbs to intensify their healing qualities.

▶ **MAGICAL POWERS:** Helps to find and keep a good sexual relationship. A protective and powerful stone, sunstone adds energy to other stones as well as to rituals and spellworkings.

MAGICAL USES

Use sunstone and moonstone as part of Solstice rituals, either on the altar or by having the priest wear the sunstone and the priestess the moonstone. This represents a balance of power between the physical attributes and the psychic, spiritual ones.

Sunstone can also be added to herbs to strengthen them. It can be kept with candles and other ritual supplies for the same purpose.

Tanzanite

▶ **HARDNESS:** 6.5

▶ **COLORS:** Pale bluish violet to bluish purple.

▶ **SOURCES:** Tanzania and Kenya.

▶ **FACTS:** Tanzanite, colored by the presence of vanadium, is a member of the zoisite family of minerals. These crystals have a distinct property known as pleochroism, meaning that they can appear in more than one color when viewed from different angles. Tanzanite can be seen as purple, gray, or blue. When seen in incandescent light, the stones will appear more violet. They have very few, if any, inclusions. This stone can be found in both transparent and chatoyant varieties. In one direction, tanzanite will appear as blue, in another violet. Before being heated to bring out its beautiful violet color, this stone is an unappealing yellow or brown. It should never be cleaned in ultrasonic cleaners.

▶ **HISTORY AND FOLKLORE:** None known. This gemstone, also known as lavender zoisite, was first discovered in the foothills of Mount Kilamanjaro in Tanzania, Africa, in 1967. Henry B. Platt, vice president of Tiffany's, which had exclusive rights to sell the stone, named this stone after the country of its origin. However, they are now available elsewhere. A very beautiful, delicately tinted stone, tanzanite will no longer be available when the major mines in Tanzania are depleted, and they are nearly exhausted. This gemstone comes almost exclusively from Tanzania, and the quantities are very limited. The price is reasonable if you shop around.

Both yellow and green zoisite have been found in Tanzania and Kenya, but their gem quality is not that of tanzanite.

Some writers associate this stone with the sign of Virgo.

To dream of tanzanite symbolizes a period of quiet and calm.

▶ **HEALING ENERGIES:** Unknown.

▶ **MAGICAL POWERS:** Very balancing for highly active people; mellows out extremes in a personality. Helps in understanding why things are happening in life by calming and balancing emotions.

Excellent for meditation as it increases spiritual awareness. Makes one sensitive to psychic experiences. When using this stone, be certain your motives are positive or you will incur negative karma.

MAGICAL USES

Wearing jewelry that contains tanzanite helps to take the edge off emotional experiences. Be aware, however, that at the same time it will make you more sensitive to spirit messages and psychic happenings.

Tektites: see Meteorite

Thulite

- ▶ **HARDNESS:** 6.5
- ▶ **COLOR:** Pale pink to raspberry red.
- ▶ **SOURCE:** Norway, Austria, western Australia, Italy, and North Carolina.
- ▶ **FACTS:** A massive member of the zoisite family, thulite is colored by manganese. It can be confused with rhodonite, because of its coloring. It is usually carved and polished as small ornaments.
- ▶ **HISTORY AND FOLKLORE:** This stone was first described in 1903 and is named after the old title of Scandinavia, which was Thule. Thulite, especially from Norway, was used primarily as a stone for carvings and cabochons. A member of the zoisite family, thulite is related to tanzanite.

  Thulite can be connected with Pisces and Gemini.

  To dream of this stone means you need to truthfully review your behavior. Some of your actions are alienating other people.
- ▶ **HEALING ENERGIES:** Unknown.
- ▶ **MAGICAL POWERS:** Helps with avoiding extremes in attitudes and behavior, such as bossiness, overextending of self, and martyr complex.

MAGICAL USES

When doing past-life meditations, thulite can keep you in touch with reality, so that you do not embroider the truth about what your past lives were actually like. This stone works well with other past-life stones.

Tiger's-Eye

▶ **HARDNESS:** 7

▶ **COLORS:** Black with yellow and golden brown.

▶ **SOURCES:** South Africa, the U.S.

▶ **FACTS:** Tiger's-eye is a variety of chalcedony or quartz with silky chatoyancy, or cat's-eye properties. Tiger's-eye has a black background with iron oxide staining that produces the yellow and golden brown striping for which this stone is known.

▶ **HISTORY AND FOLKLORE:** This stone has been worn for centuries as protection against the evil eye and spells.

Tiger's-eye is often associated with the signs of Capricorn and Leo.

To dream of this stone symbolizes a need to keep alert; something or someone is hiding the truth behind a veil of illusion.

▶ **HEALING ENERGIES:** Helpful to the spleen, pancreas, and digestive organs. Red tiger's-eye is useful in slowing down the third chakra and flushing out excess energy. Said to be very helpful against hypochondria and psychosomatic illnesses.

▶ **MAGICAL POWERS:** Another cat's-eye stone, tiger's-eye is an emotional balancer that softens stubbornness and gives clear insight. It grounds and centers, thus strengthening the connection with the will and personal power. Balances male and female energies.

A good-luck stone, tiger's-eye is also used for discerning the truth in any situation. Can help with understanding any cycle through which one is going.

Helps one to gain greater spiritual understanding by developing inner strength and responsibility. Can defeat negative forces of all kinds. Also enhances psychic abilities. Can be used for seeing into both the past and the future.

This stone focuses the power of the mind in such a way that an all-seeing mental "eye" is created.

Use when trying to determine karmic ties and past-life connections with family, friends, or acquaintances.

MAGICAL USES

If you sincerely desire to know the truth about family past-life connections, put several pieces of tumbled tiger's-eye around the divination area when you cast runes or read cards. If you scry into the past, put a tiger's-eye with your scrying ball or mirror for seven days before you try.

Wear or carry this stone for protection. It is especially good against all kinds of dark magic.

Titanite

▶ **HARDNESS:** 5
▶ **COLORS:** Yellow, green, brown, other colors.
▶ **SOURCES:** Austria, Canada, Switzerland, Madagascar, Mexico, and Brazil.
▶ **FACTS:** Also known as sphene, titanite has a very strong fire, even higher than diamond. It also is pleochroic (showing three colors at once) and doubling of an image when looked through.
▶ **HISTORY AND FOLKLORE:** None known.

Titanite can be associated with the signs of Virgo and Cancer.

To dream of this stone means a coming period of feeling bound and restricted.
▶ **HEALING ENERGIES:** Unknown.
▶ **MAGICAL POWERS:** Helpful to those who work in areas that demand compassion, such as hospitals, nursing homes, or with mentally disturbed people. It is also helpful to those who must care for sick or disturbed family members.

MAGICAL USES

Keep a piece of tumbled or polished titanite as a small touchstone. When you feel overwhelmed by the emotions connected with your profession or duties, spend a few minutes holding this stone. Because it does absorb nervous energy as well as exude calming vibrations, you will need to cleanse the titanite frequently.

Topaz

▶ **HARDNESS:** 8

▶ **COLORS:** A range of colors, including white, pale blue, green, pink, and through shades of yellow-brown.

▶ **SOURCES:** Minas Gerais, Brazil, southern California, Sri Lanka, Myanmar, the Ural Mountains of Russia, Australia, Tasmania, Pakistan, Mexico, Japan, Cornwall, England, and Zimbabwe, Nigeria, and southwest Africa. Topaz crystals are also found in the Mountains of Mourne in Ireland.

▶ **FACTS:** The word topaz comes from the Sanskrit word *tapas* or *topas* ("fire"). Topaz is made up of hard, pyramid-topped crystals and belongs to the orthorhombic system. There are several different colors, each with its own unique refractive qualities. The topaz has a similar specific gravity to diamond, although the way it disperses light and sparkle is much lower than diamond. A few topaz stones have tear-shaped interior inclusions containing gas bubbles or liquids.

Good-quality gemstones up to 35,000 carats have been faceted. In 1940, a New York gem dealer purchased three specimens of topaz from Brazil, one weighing 596 pounds, another 300 pounds, and the third 225 pounds. Blue topaz has the same specific gravity and refraction as the colorless stones and is often mistaken for aquamarine. The yellow, brown, and pink topaz have a lower specific gravity and a higher refraction than the colorless and blue ones. However, it is the golden yellow topaz (sometimes called sherry) that most represents this stone.

The Imperial, or sherry yellow, topaz is the most valuable, especially the medium to large specimens. In its crystalline form, the longer, uncut stones are slightly darker at the ends. Most of it comes from Brazil, but small amounts are also found in Russia, Japan, Sri Lanka, Burma, Germany, and the United States.

True red and pink topaz are rarely found, although a very few have been discovered in Pakistan. Pink topaz can range from yellowish pink or orange-pink to medium pink tending to a red or violet tinge. Pink topaz mainly comes from Brazil and the Ural Mountains in Russia. Almost all of the pink topaz usually sold today is actually heat-treated brown. The process for obtaining this salmon pink color was discovered in 1750 by a Parisian jeweler. This process began, and continued, because the intense colors were more valuable than the paler stones.

Colorless, transparent topaz is found in Brazil, Russia, Germany, the United States, Japan, Nigeria, Zaire, and Namibia. Because of its low value, it is often treated to become a specific color. Some of these are quite popular, such as the Swiss Blue (an icy blue) and the London Blue (a richer, deeper shade of blue). The colorless topaz that is used to make London Blue is irradiated, producing a beautiful dark blue; this may soon be extremely rare if the procedure is halted, which is likely. White topaz was also known as the Slave's Diamond at one time.

Natural blue topaz ranges from a uniform sky blue to the rare intense blue. It is mined in Brazil, Mexico, the United States, Burma, Russia, Namibia, and Nigeria. It is the least expensive of all topaz.

What is called Oriental Topaz is not topaz at all, but either citrine or yellow sapphire, while amethyst that has been heat-treated is sold as Madeira topaz. Most of the yellow-brown or sherry-colored topaz on the market today is sold as Scottish topaz, although it actually comes from South America. Reputable gem traders will call this yellow topaz Brazilian topaz, however. Both smoky quartz and citrine are often presented as topaz.

▶ **HISTORY AND FOLKLORE:** The golden topaz was not known by that name to the ancient cultures, which classed all golden, transparent stones as "Chrysolite"; this name also covered all yellow-green stones and the green peridot. The name Chrysolite may have come from the Greek words *kreusos* ("gold") and *lithos* ("stone") or the Latin words *crisos* ("gold") and *oletus* ("whole"), which would mean "wholly gold." This stone was dedicated to Apollo, the Sun deity.

Ancient manuscripts say that the finest chrysolites were exclusively found on an island called Serpent Isle, located in the Red Sea. Pliny knew of this island under the name of *Topazos* ("to conjecture"); however, the stones mined there were peridots, not topaz.

Pliny wrote that the powers of this stone increased as the Moon increased. Calling it the "stone of strength," he and other ancient writers believed that topaz lost its color in the presence of poison, could give one glimpses of the future by strengthening ties with the astral world, and protected against epidemics.

Saffron yellow topaz has always been popular in India, where it is worn for health, wisdom, and to prevent sudden death. Ancient members of ruling royalty wore topaz to attract riches and power. The Romans wore yellow topaz as protection when traveling, to bring riches and favors, and to prevent burns.

Many physicians of the fourth, fifth, and sixth centuries believed that the topaz exuded a milky fluid on occasion; this fluid was considered to be an antidote for rabies. Roman physicians said that the touch of chrysolite (topaz) should be used to treat the plague and serious skin diseases; this belief was still held by the Bishop of Renness in 1081. Strung on a donkey's hair, topaz was said to guard against evil spirits and nightmares. Even Albertus Magnus (1193–1280) wrote that the topaz was useful to treat hemorrhoids, bleeding wounds, gout, insanity, excessive anger, and epilepsy. Like many other stones, topaz also protected against enchantments and illusions. During the Middle Ages, St. Hildegarde, Abbess of Bingen, devised an eye lotion that was said to cure failing eyesight. She steeped topaz in wine for three days and night, then lightly touched the eyeball with the solution.

The ancient Greeks also used topaz in the end of long wands that they used as divining rods to find gold and other precious metals.

When a thunderstorm approaches, topaz is said to become very strongly electric in nature. This action tends to make the wearer restless and causes clairvoyant visions.

Topaz is sometimes connected with the sign of Sagittarius.

To dream of topaz predicts protection and movement in your affairs.

▶ **HEALING ENERGIES:** Helpful in treating high blood pressure; reduces varicose veins. Helps the blood and circulation in general.

Said to also relieve depression and arthritis, as well as help the digestive system.

Blue: This color of the stone also aids in regeneration of tissue as well as strengthening the thyroid gland and enhancing the metabolism.

Gold: Can detoxify the body and help with tissue regeneration. Strengthens the digestive organs and nervous system. It can also help in nervous trauma, mental confusion, and exhaustion. Place on the bodies of the dying to help them gain a peaceful transition.

▶ **MAGICAL POWERS:** Dispels nightmares and contagion; helps with predictive dreams. Also aids with messages from the astral. Guards against depression and negativity by creating a spirit of hope. Makes sound, dreamless sleep possible. Makes one more aware and open to creative thinking. Said to prevent accidents and fires. Especially good to repel envy, intrigue, injury, sudden death, and negative magic. Use in combination with tiger's-eye when working spells for wealth.

Blue: Its cool, soothing, tranquil vibrations help to balance the emotions. It helps with healing, creativity, self-expression, and psychic perception. Also aids with communing with the Higher Self and spirit guides. Those who work in creative fields will find this helpful for inspiration.

Clear: opens communication with non-human species.

Gold and yellow: Ruled by the Sun. Brings abundance; encourages practicality and good planning. Worn on the left hand or arm, the topaz is said to prevent sleepwalking, calm anger, heal the mind, and repel enchantments. A stone that has more power at night than during daylight hours, it will protect the house against fire and burglars, and the wearer against accidents. One of the luckiest of stones, it will attract wealth and helpful friends.

Green: helps to keep one from adding to karma by heavy thoughts of revenge.

Imperial (sherry-colored): helpful to scholars and students; encourages the seeking and retaining of knowledge. This color of topaz has a stimulating effect on the higher mind, charging the aura with greater awareness, concentration, clarity of vision, and creativity. Old sources also say it helps to give a painless death.

Pink: encourages integrity and honesty.

White: stimulates the mind for better intellectual focus. Has much the same effect as amber, but is not as powerful.

MAGICAL USES

Use a piece of yellow topaz with a tiger's-eye and both a green and a yellow candle in a regular candle-burning ritual for prosperity. Write out on a small paper the high points of what you consider as prosperity. If you believe your prosperity will come through your job, add a white topaz for focused thinking. After the candles have burned completely out, wrap the stones in the paper and tie with green thread. Sleep with them under your pillow for seven days. Then remove the stones and burn the paper.

Tourmaline

▶ **HARDNESS:** 7
▶ **COLORS:** Many colors.
▶ **SOURCES:** (Rubellite) Russia, the U.S., Madagascar, Brazil, Myanmar, and East Africa. (Indicolite) Siberia, Brazil, Madagascar, and the U.S. (Dravite) Sri Lanka, the U.S., Canada, Mexico, Brazil, and Australia. (Achroite) Madagascar and the U.S. (Watermelon) South Africa, Brazil, East Africa, and others. (Schorl) Worldwide. (Yellow and Green) Brazil, Tanzania, Namibia, and Sri Lanka.
▶ **FACTS:** The name tourmaline comes from the Sinhalese word *turmali* or *toramalli*, which refers to gems of unknown identity. In eighteenth century England, the word tourmaline was written as tumalin.

Tourmaline is often confused with other precious gems because of its great variety of colors. It has the greatest range of colors of all gemstones: colorless, pink, green, blue, brown, and all intermediate hues. There is also an unusual purple color that comes from the Ural Mountains in Russia and is called siberite.

There are tourmalines that have two or more colors, such as the watermelon tourmaline from Brazil. The mines of Mozambique, Angola, Tanzania, and Zambia also produce a tourmaline that is the reverse of the watermelon: green center with pink around it. Red tourmaline is also known as elbaite.

Brazil also mines an intense green tourmaline called the Brazilian Emerald; another name for this stone is chrome green tourmaline. This particular tourmaline was, and is, often mistaken by the general public for the emerald. At one time, the Brazilian Emerald was set in episcopal rings.

Achroite tourmaline is a rare, colorless member of this stone group. Its name comes from the Greek word *achroos*, which means without color. It is often heat-treated to produce pale pink stones.

Dravite tourmaline is rich in magnesium; this produces a very dark brown, orange-brown, or golden brown color. This particular variety will appear colored in one direction and colorless in another. Sometimes it is heat-treated to lighten the color if the stone is considered too dark. The name comes from the Drave district in Austria.

The dark blue tourmaline is called indicolite, or sometimes indigolite. It can also be greenish blue and indigo. Indicolite can appear green or blue in one direction, with a loss of transparency in the other. The most important source of this color is Siberia, Russia, where the lilac to violet blue to violet red variety is known as siberite. Bright blue tourmaline is mined in Paraiba, Brazil. Other sources are Colorado, Massachusetts, California, Namibia, and Madagascar.

Rubellite, from the Latin word for red, is actually many shades of pink, violet pink, or red. The ruby red stones are the most valuable. Some rubellite has fibrous inclusions, which produce a cat's-eye effect when cut *en cabochon*. Rubellite is found in Russia, Burma, Sri Lanka, Brazil, California, and Madagascar.

Black tourmaline, also known as schorl, is the most common and widely distributed, although it is not considered to have value as a gem.

Yellow, yellow-green, and green are the most common colors of tourmaline, with the green color range going from bright green to olivine to yellow-green. However, the deep emerald green is quite rare and very valuable. This color is found in Brazil, Maine, Tanzania, Mozambique, Namibia, Russia, and Sri Lanka.

▶ **HISTORY AND FOLKLORE:** This stone has been used for over 2000 years. The Romans and Greeks apparently imported tourmaline from the Orient, for a ring of the second or third century has an inscription identifying its origin as India.

Tourmaline has been used in jewelry in the Middle and Far East for centuries, but it was not until the Dutch colonists introduced it to Europe about 1700 that this stone became widely known. At first, the Dutch only used the long tourmaline crystals to clean ash from pipes. Because of this use, the Dutch called tourmaline *ashentrekker* or Ash Puller. After 1750, when the stone was very popular, it became known by the Sinhalese name of *toramalli*. The Germans knew it as *azchenzieher* and the French as *tire-cendre*. As far back as ancient Rome, Pliny called this stone *lychnis*.

Somewhat like amber, tourmaline is pyroelectric, developing an electrical charge if it is heated. The Swedish scholar Linnaeus referred to this stone as the "electric stone." Tourmaline also develops piezoelectricity when placed under stress. These two qualities brought about the use of tourmaline in thermometers and depth and pressure gauges. When a slice is cut from the length of a prism face, tourmaline will polarize light. Despite this stone being both pyroelectric and piezoelectric, it is a nonconductor of electricity. Unlike topaz, tourmaline will float in water.

Some writers associate this stone with Libra.

To dream of tourmaline means to be watchful of unexpected and potential dangers.

▶ **HEALING ENERGIES:** A Gemini stone, tourmaline is occasionally found in the form of wands. Highly prized as healing tools, these wands channel powerful energies that can do great healings. It is also believed that knowledgeable magicians can do miracles with these wands.

Verdelite (green): heals on all levels. Strengthens and purifies the nervous system.

Watermelon: excellent for harmonizing the energies in the heart and nervous system. All tourmaline can affect the nervous system. A powerful healer because of its highly electromagnetic energy field.

▶ MAGICAL POWERS: All colors of tourmaline have many of the same qualities, although different colors will affect different chakras. Use tourmaline along with such stones as malachite to connect the upper chakras with the lower ones, thus getting your energy flow into the correct rhythm.

Can build up and maintain a powerful personal protection shield, as well as self-assurance. A prime protection stone, tourmaline can ward off fear and negativity, while inspiring self-confidence and understanding.

Helps to balance the endocrine system and revitalizes the body and mind. Can aid in sleep. By activating certain vibrations of the body and mind, this stone aligns the subtle bodies and gives a strong protective influence. Breaks up and removes fear and negative conditions; a strong protector.

By enhancing sensitivity and understanding, it helps with concentration and inspiration. A stone that inspires creativity, tourmaline is very helpful to artists, writers, actors, musicians, and others in the fields of the arts.

Helps in being flexible and less emotionally involved in charged issues; yet it also causes one to be more objective in purpose.

Tourmaline wands are extremely powerful but also very expensive. Because they are rarely placed on the market, these wands can easily cost several hundred dollars. They come in either solid or in graduating colors and can be up to eight inches long. Power channeled through these wands is intensified to a high vibration.

Achroite (rare and colorless): helps with clear seeing in everyday events and in foretelling.

Blue-green: helps in opening the life to new friends and new experiences.

Buergerite (iridescent dark brown): basically has the same energies as dravite.

Chromdravite (dark green): attracts money and business success.

Dravite (very dark brown, orange-brown, or golden brown): balances the fifth chakra; aids in intellectual processing.

Indicolite (blue): gives calmness, clarity of insight. Teaches spiritual Oneness.

Rubellite and elbaite (red, dark pink): sometimes called the queen of the tourmalines, it relaxes and calms. Aids in directing spiritual urges and desires. Helps to soften grief and inner pain caused by conflicts. A heart chakra stone, it helps to release deeply buried emotional experiences. Works well with rose quartz and kunzite. Helps to release past sorrows over love and prepare to love again.

Schorl (black): heals houseplants. Strengthens astral travel, processing of information from past lives, and transformation of the self to a higher level. Aids in understanding abstract ideas. Deflects negativity and can be used as a protective shield that will deflect all physical and psychic negative energies. Changes and releases internal negativity. Can cause vibrations or events to slow down so that one can assess things better. When found inside clear quartz crystal, schorl is called tourmalinated quartz.

Siberite (lilac to violet purple): aids in opening the intuition and psychic senses.

Tsilaisite (yellow and brown): helps strengthen the mind when studying or researching; also aids in contact with etheric Otherworld beings.

Verdelite (green to dark green): aids with communications. Helps in seeking wisdom from Nature and Nature spirits. A regenerating stone, it can realign the bodies after shattering experiences. Attracts prosperity and inspires creative ideas. Aids in working through a problem to the end. Can help in recognizing and avoiding negative energies.

Watermelon (pink and green): helps one stick to a task until it is finished. Excellent for removing imbalances and guilt, conflicts and confusion. A problem-solving stone, watermelon tourmaline helps one to accept the past and plan for a better future.

Yellow: balances the fifth chakra; strengthens the intellect.

MAGICAL USES

Tourmaline can be purchased shaped into balls, pyramids, pillars, or wands. A wonderful and versatile stone, it can be used in most rituals and spellworkings without upsetting the energy balance of other stones present. If you handle your pieces of tourmaline often, they become extremely sensitive to your vibrations and rapidly respond to whatever you are doing.

Turquoise

► **HARDNESS:** 5–6
► **COLORS:** Sky blue to blue-white, light green-blue to light green; usually opaque.
► **SOURCES:** Iran, Pakistan, Tibet, Mexico, the U.S., Russia, Chile, Australia, Turkestan, and Cornwall.
► **FACTS:** A massive stone, not a crystal, turquoise has long been mined, used, and prized by cultures around the world. It is opaque to semi-translucent and very fragile. It can easily fade or crack.

Turquoise got its name from the Turkish merchants who first carried this stone to Europe for trading. Turquoise was first exported to Germany where they were known as *Turkisher steins* ("Turkish stones"). The French translated this into *Pierre turquoise* ("stone of Turkey"). This stone was known to the Venetians as *turchesa*, to the Germans as *turkis*, to the Tibetans as *gyu*, to the Chinese as *yu*, to the Mexicans as *chalchihuitl*, and to the Persians as *Piruzeh* ("the Triumphant"). An ancient Egyptian name for this stone was *majkat*; they mined it at *Serabit el Khadim* near the temple of the goddess Hathor, who was called Goddess of Turquoise.[61]

Turquoise is primarily noted for its beautiful blue color, which many think is produced by copper, ammonium, and traces of iron. The blue color ranges from the most-sought sky blue to a bluish green. The finest sky blue turquoise is mined in Iran.

The color of turquoise can be greatly affected by a number of things: acid perspiration that can turn the stone green; too much warmth; the alcohol in perfumes, hair spray, and cosmetics. The Arabs say that turquoise is so sensitive to atmospheric conditions that its color is affected by changes in weather. This belief of the connection of weather and turquoise is also known to the Orientals, and the Pueblo and Apache Indians.

▶ **HISTORY AND FOLKLORE:** The Egyptians mined turquoise in the Sinai Peninsula from earliest times. The Persians of present-day Iran also mined this stone, for there are recovered beads dating from c. 5000 B.C.E. The best turquoise still comes from Iran. This stone was also used in Siberian jewelry dating back to the fifth century B.C.E.

The early Egyptians knew of this stone and mined it. Their goddess Isis was called Lady of the Turquoise,[62] although there is some dispute as to whether the stone meant is lapis lazuli or turquoise. Pliny later called it by the name of *callais*. Highly prized as an amulet, the Turks called turquoise by the name *Fayruz*, "the lucky stone." This stone may be identical to the Moslem *sakhrat*, a sacred stone that was taken from Mount Qaf, which was itself the habitation of fairies.

According to thirteenth-century records, the Turks attached turquoise to horse bridles to protect both the horse and rider from falls and injuries; this practice probably dates back even further than the records show. By the beginning of the seventeenth century in Europe, turquoise was well-known, held in high regard, and worn by men; it was unusual for a woman to wear turquoise.

Turquoise was known and used by the Aztecs, Toltecs, and Olmecs for centuries. The Aztecs got their supply from Mount Chalchihuitl in Cerrillos, New Mexico, where mining was begun about a thousand years ago. Some of their most magnificent artifacts are the death masks inlaid with turquoise mosaic. No one was allowed to wear this stone, for it was used only as an offering to the gods. After the conquest and destruction of the Mayan Empire by Cortez in 1533 C.E., the reverence for turquoise was held only by the Pueblo people of the Southwest and the Apache. The Apache knew this stone as *duklij*. Among the Apaches, every medicine man had to have a piece of turquoise, or he was considered to have no power or respect. A holy stone, turquoise was sometimes thrown into rivers to bring rain.

Universally known as the Venus stone, turquoise is another stone credited with the power to turn aside the evil eye. Even today, many people in the Middle East wear turquoise beads or tie them in the manes and tails of camels, mules, and oxen for good luck and to assure that the animals do not fall down and injure themselves. From about the thirteenth century this idea was prevalent all over Europe, not only of turquoise protecting the horse, but the rider or any wearer from severe injury as well. It was thought that the turquoise bead or ring attracted to itself the force of the fall or blow and would crack, rather than the wearer come to harm.

Turquoise was part of the medical equipment of most physicians of the fifteenth century; they claimed that this stone would counteract the effects of any poison. They also powdered the stone in a potion as a cure for scorpion stings and pains caused by the possession by demons. Placing turquoise on the eyes or looking at it was said to relieve eyestrain. If the wearer of a turquoise became ill, the stone was thought to turn pale; if the wearer died, the turquoise was said to lose all its color until possessed by a new, healthy wearer. The Czar Ivan the Terrible of Russia firmly believed this, as recorded by one of Elizabeth I's messengers.

The ancient Persians knew of other magical uses of turquoise. They said if the stone was a dazzling blue in the morning, it foretold of a happy, fine day. A Persian spell for good fortune and the repulsion of evil said one had to see the reflection of the New Moon on a turquoise or a copy of the Koran.

Both Native Americans and Tibetan Buddhists hold turquoise in the highest regard, saying that it gives life and breath to the Earth and its creatures, and that it is one of the protectors and guardians of the body and soul. Both cultures combine turquoise with red coral, symbol of the life-force.

Turquoise is considered to be a symbol of generosity, sincerity, and affection. It preserves friendships and can make friends out of enemies. Traditionally it is said to only bring good luck if given, not bought. However, this is not always true; the innate energy of each stone must be considered separately.

Turquoise is often associated with Venus and the signs of Sagittarius, Pisces, and Scorpio.

If you see a turquoise in your dreams, it foretells prosperity.

► **HEALING ENERGIES:** A master healer and a stone of yin ("feminine") energy, turquoise helps with female disorders. Also used to prevent and cure headaches. Said to lose its color when the wearer is under great stress. A strong stone for toning and strengthening the entire body and regenerating tissue, turquoise also aids in improving circulation and correcting any problems with the circulation and respiratory systems. Tradition says this stone reflects the health of the body and aura by changing color.

► **MAGICAL POWERS:** Enhances meditation by helping with creativity, peace of mind, communication, and emotional balance. A protecting and balancing stone, turquoise can align the chakras. Helps to reconcile friends and lovers. Gently urges the wearer to seek out answers and knowledge.

Called "skystone" or "stone of heaven" by some Native Americans, the vibrations of turquoise can build a spiritual bridge between worlds and give strong psychic powers.

To gain prosperity, hold a piece of turquoise in the right hand and speak your wishes directly into the stone while looking at it steadily.

MAGICAL USES

Turquoise beads are excellent for hanging in the car for protection. They can also be attached inconspicuously to your key chain, purse, lapel, or even the baby stroller. The blue bead to turn aside the evil eye and negative magic is still widely used throughout the Middle East.

Vanadinite

► **HARDNESS:** 2.5–3
► **COLORS:** orange-red, scarlet red, and brown-yellow.

▶ **SOURCES:** Morocco, Mexico, the U.S., and South Africa.

▶ **FACTS:** Vanadinite is so very similar to pryomorphite and mimetite in its color ranges and structure that it is difficult to identify from the others without chemical analysis. Generally, its prismatic crystals are small with central cavities and rounded edges; sometimes it forms very beautiful druses with tiny crystals. Lead contributes to its mineral composition.

▶ **HISTORY AND FOLKLORE:** None that we know of under the present name. In 1830, the Swedish chemist Nils Sefstrom named this mineral in honor of the Norse goddess Freyja, who was also known by the title Vanadis. She was a member of the deity group called the Vanir, who were already in Asgard when Odhinn and the Aesir gods arrived.

Vanadinite can be connected with Venus and the sign of Taurus.

To dream of this mineral symbolizes a spiritual need to get closer to the Goddess and your feminine side.

▶ **HEALING ENERGIES:** Unknown.

▶ **MAGICAL POWERS:** Gives inspiration of a spiritual nature. Helps one touch the Center and become balanced.

MAGICAL USES

Usually found as crusts of small crystals, vanadinite's primary use is spiritual. Place it on the altar with flowers and green or pink candles when communicating with the Goddess. Hold a piece of vanadinite or have it nearby when meditating on spiritual paths.

Volcanic Glass (Obsidian)

▶ **HARDNESS:** 5

▶ **COLORS:** Usually black, but can be brown or gray; rare colors are red, blue, and green.

▶ **SOURCE:** Worldwide in volcanic areas.

▶ **FACTS:** A natural glass formed by volcanic action, obsidian has no cleavage. It is simply volcanic melt that cooled so fast when exposed to the air that it formed no crystals. The usual color is black, but brown and gray are also frequently found. The rare colors of red, blue, and green are seldom seen and very expensive. Obsidian may be all one color, or can be striped or spotted. A blue variety is found on the British coast, while dark brown and black obsidian, sometimes flecked with white so-called *christobalite*, are found in the Italian Lipari Islands, Iceland, and the United States. Sometimes a very rare brown obsidian with red flame markings (*bergmahonie*) is discovered.

Internal bubbles or crystals sometimes create a random pattern, such as in snowflake obsidian. Other inclusions give some obsidian a metallic or iridescent gold or silver sheen as in rainbow obsidian. Another anomaly can produce an eye-stone when the obsidian is polished into a ball. Because obsidian is fragile, it is seldom cut for jewelry.

There are other forms of obsidian that have their own names, according to the locale in which they are found. Californite (California) is green; cyprine (Norway) is blue and very rare; xanthite (New York) is yellow-green; and wiluite (Russia) is green. The dark nodules known as Apache Tears are found in Arizona and New Mexico; these are black or dark brown in color. Mount St. Helen's glass was discovered after the volcano of that name erupted in Washington State in 1980; this type of obsidian is treated to turn a dark green or teal green color. Vesuvianite, which can be red, yellow, green, brown, or purple, was first discovered on the slopes of the Italian volcano Vesuvius; sometimes it is called idocrase. Vesuvianite can be confused with some garnets, diopside, smoky quartz, tourmaline, and zircon.

▶ **HISTORY AND FOLKLORE:** Early in human history, obsidian was used to make knives, mirrors, and ornamental objects. The ancient cultures in Mexico called this stone Itzli; they got their supply from the Hill of the Knives, which is not far from Timapau. They fashioned obsidian into images of the god *Tezcatlipoca* ("shining mirror") and into magic divinatory mirrors. They knew obsidian as *iztli* or *teotetl* ("the divine stone").[63] Other Native American cultures used this stone in ceremonies to sharpen the inner sight. Obsidian vases and mirrors are often discovered in ancient Mexican graves.

The type of obsidian called Pele's Hair comes from the Hawaiian Islands and is named after the Polynesian volcanic goddess Pele. The ancient Polynesian culture believed that Pele, who kept the souls of the dead in her Underworld realm, sent them back to the Earth along with her lava, so they could be reincarnated.

The Romans and Greeks used obsidian to make cameos and other jewelry. The Roman Pliny wrote that obsidian got its name from a man called Obsidius, who discovered it in Ethiopia.

The famous Dr. John Dee, who was magician-alchemist to Queen Elizabeth I of England, was said to have had an obsidian scrying mirror.

Some writers associate obsidian with the sign of Sagittarius. Others say obsidian is a Saturn stone, while others place it with Pluto. Some say the snowflake obsidian is connected with Virgo.

To dream of obsidian in any color means a period of darkness and struggle will soon be ended.

▶ **HEALING ENERGIES:** Aids the stomach and intestines. A powerful healer stone but only for some magicians. Helps to improve the vision.

▶ **MAGICAL POWERS:** By grounding spiritual energy in the physical plane, it connects the mind and emotions. Absorbs and destroys negative energies, thus clearing subconscious blockages and reducing stress. Helps to understand and use the state of detachment. Can bring an understanding of the deep silence and wisdom found in meditation. Protects from evil spirits; aids in developing clairvoyance. Use to draw the aura more tightly about the body and regroup your scattered energies.

A scrying ball of black obsidian is extremely powerful and should be used with caution. If its energy and intenseness makes you uncomfortable, hold a clear quartz crystal in one hand while scrying.

Obsidian is also helpful in understanding, dealing with, and balancing the negative and positive cycles in life. Its power can be blunt as it brings up the unvarnished dark areas of the subconscious that need changing before one can advance. Helps grief by absorbing the grieving energies, transforming them into positive spiritual lessons.

Black obsidian is one of the most difficult stones to use if you are not prepared to face reality, both positive and negative. Since it energizes spiritual forces and easily connects with the first chakra, black obsidian can make you face present challenges and past-life lessons still to be learned. The third eye is often activated in connection with processing of past-life karma—positive or negative. It is often best used along with clear quartz.

Black, brown, or golden: aids in eliminating bad habits; reduces cravings.

Mahogany: makes one feel sexier and more at ease with one's sensuality.

Rainbow: balances and stabilizes energy; good for calming fears after any abusive situation; helps to balance mental distress. Its relaxing, balancing effect aids in using creativity.

Silver or gold sheen: stimulates activity and health.

Snowflake (black and gray): helps one slow down and balance activities. Helps one to think more clearly and logically. Keep a piece with your money to keep it from running out. Carry snowflake obsidian to keep people from taking advantage of you. Snowflake obsidian will also reveal what needs to be changed within your life, so you can advance.

Vesuvianite (dark brown-green): gives you the energy for competing, but without the arrogance and cruelty so often involved.

MAGICAL USES

Obsidian is excellent just to have around to absorb and transform negative energies, give off vibrations of calmness and security, and stabilize the energies of all persons within its reach. People are fascinated by obsidian and like to pick it up and run their fingers over it. One of the few stones that absorb negative vibrations without storing them, volcanic glass makes a wonderful desk or coffee table ornament. If you have cats and/or small children, be prepared to wipe off finger and nose prints; it seems to give off an aura of "please touch me."

To keep money from running through your fingers, put a small piece of obsidian in your wallet with the paper money.

Apache Tear

▶ **COLORS:** Black or dark brown.

▶ **HISTORY AND FOLKLORE:** The name of this stone comes from a legend of the Apache. After a great defeat in battle and the death of many brave warriors, the Apache women mourned over the bodies. Their tears solidified and turned into this stone. It is said that anyone who has an Apache Tear will never cry again.

▶ **HEALING ENERGIES:** Unknown.

▶ **MAGICAL POWERS:**

Apache Gold (black with metallic gold streaks): aids in slowing down; similar to pyrite.

Apache Tears: good for channeling spirit guides and higher beings; creates harmony, balance, and moderation. Excellent for increasing psychic powers. Also attracts success in any business venture.

MAGICAL USES

The small pieces of obsidian known as Apache Tears are very good to hold or wear during meditations to contact your spirit guides. One woman I know has a special pair of earrings with Apache Tears, which she wears only when meditating or trancing. She says that since earrings are close to both the sixth and seventh chakras, any stones set in them work directly on these psychic centers. My own experiments with this idea has proved productive.

Mount Saint Helens Glass

▶ **COLORS:** teal green, teal blue, deep blue, rose pink.

▶ **SOURCE:** Mount Saint Helens, Washington State.

▶ **FACTS:** After Mount Saint Helens erupted in May 1980, rocks and ash were found on its slopes that had come from miles below, within the volcano. Certain people found that they could use debris from the volcanic eruption of this mountain to produce beautiful translucent stones. Very similar to other volcanic glass, these stones are manmade, although they are composed of volcanic materials.

▶ **HISTORY AND FOLKLORE:** None.

▶ **HEALING ENERGIES:** Unknown.

▶ **MAGICAL POWERS:** Attracts business and career success. However, if properly accessed, the vibrations of this type of volcanic glass cause events to happen rapidly, so be prepared.

MAGICAL USES

To connect with the vibrations of Mount Saint Helens glass you will have to spend some time handling, wearing, and contemplating this stone. It seems that over a period of time your vibrations and those of the stone gradually match, and this appears to set up the psychic and astral connections. I purchased a ring set with this stone and at first found nothing much emanating from it. However, over a period of time as I worked with it, the energies became more apparent and powerful. When I wore it during ritual and spellworking, events worked for came very fast. If you are the more leisurely paced person, you will probably be uncomfortable with this stone.

Wulfenite

▶ **HARDNESS:** 2.5–3

▶ **COLOR:** Reddish orange, orange, and yellow.

▶ **SOURC.E.:** Arizona, Morocco, Mexico, the Congo, Algeria, Namibia, and Australia.

▶ **FACTS:** A colorful lead molybdate mineral that is found in the oxide zones of many old copper, lead, and silver mines. It is often found with vanadinite, cerussite, pyromorphite, and mimetite. Its crystals are quite beautiful, differently unique, and very heavy. Also known as the butterscotch stone, it is usually found in shiny tabular crystals that resemble butterscotch candy. The rare fiery red wulfenite crystals are mined in the Red Cloud mine in Arizona.

▶ **HISTORY AND FOLKLORE:** No ancient history that we know of under the present name. Wulfenite was named in honor of the Austrian mineralogist Franz Xavier von Wulfen (1728–1805).

Wulfenite can be associated with Mars and the signs of Aries, Taurus, and Scorpio.

To dream of this stone symbolizes a deep need for relaxation and contact with Nature.

▶ **HEALING ENERGIES:** Unknown.

▶ **MAGICAL POWERS:** Helps in communication with Nature spirits and devas; also helps in connecting with the forces of Nature, such as plants, water, air currents, etc.

MAGICAL USES

Set wulfenite on your altar along with gingerroot to attract Nature spirits and those connected with the elements. Meditating with this stone will aid you in making stronger contact with these Otherworld beings and enlisting their help in projects.

Zircon

▶ **HARDNESS:** 6–7.5

▶ **COLORS:** Colorless, yellow, orange, brown, blue, red, green.

▶ **SOURCES:** Sri Lanka, Myanmar, Thailand, Cambodia, Vietnam, Kampuchea, Australia, Brazil, Nigeria, Tanzania, and France.

▶ **FACTS:** Zircon looks much like diamond and in the past has been both mistaken for diamond and intentionally sold as such. The difference lies in the double refraction and the wear on its softer edges of the facet. Brown zircon comes from Thailand, Vietnam, and Kampuchea; these are usually heat-treated to produce colorless or blue stones, both colors being popular for jewelry. The name zircon comes from the Arabic word *zargun* ("gold color").

The stone known in old records as the jargoon is actually a colorless or white zircon, while hyacinth and jacinth (ruled by Mars) refer to deep orange or rich red zircon. Jacinth is a name of Arabic origin, while hyacinth comes from Greek. The actual name zircon may have come from the Arabic word *zirk* ("a jewel"). In ancient Sanskrit writings, this stone is known as *Rahuratna*, or stones of the Nodes of the Moon.

Colorless zircon often has a slight gray or smoky tinge; it is brittle and the edges of faceted stones easily damage. In the past these stones were known as Matara diamonds, from the city at the tip of Sri Lanka, the country that is renowned for colorless zircons. In old records, most writers say this color of zircon was called a jargoon, which may come from either the Persian word *zargon* or the Italian word *giacone*. Others say the yellow or orange-yellow zircon is the jargoon and is ruled by the Sun. During the Middle Ages, this stone was used as a talisman against plagues. This color of zircon is also found in Thailand and South Vietnam.

Blue zircon, also called starlite, is a light electric blue that looks green in one direction. It can also be a soft pale blue, light greenish blue, or sky blue. The electric blue stones are the most valuable. Blue zircon is mined in Cambodia, Vietnam, and Thailand.

Red zircon, once called hyacinth, can be brick red, orange-red, or violet red. This color of stone comes mainly from Sri Lanka, Cambodia, and Thailand.

Yellow zircon can vary from pale yellow to canary yellow, gold, or greenish yellow. It is found in Sri Lanka and Cambodia.

Green zircon has less luster than other zircons; it comes in colors ranging from a slightly brownish green to a cold green. Most green zircons come from Sri Lanka, while the slightly green to brownish green stones come from Burma. They are the least expensive of the zircons.

Found in Burma, Vietnam, Cambodia, and Sri Lanka, the brown zircon varies from a shade the color of black tea to reddish brown, and yellow-brown.

▶ **HISTORY AND FOLKLORE:** This stone was used in Greece and Italy as far back as the sixth century C.E. However, the earlier Hindu writings list zircon as one of the many gems on the Kalpa Tree[64] of their religion; green zircon was this mystical tree's foliage.

Zircon was said to give the wearer wisdom, honor, and riches, while the loss of its luster predicted danger. This stone was also carried by travelers to protect against accident or injury and avoid lightning strikes.

The hyacinth or jacinth was believed to drive away evil spirits and nightmares, protect from enchantment and lightning, strengthen the heart, bring sleep, and banish depression and grief. In India, it was said to attract riches, honor, and wisdom, as well as drive away evil spirits and protect from thieves. During the Middle Ages, jacinth was used to attract success and prevent from fevers and plague. In fact, it was believed that if one had a contagious disease, the jacinth's color would change when touched by that person. Paracelsus wrote that holding a jacinth against the forehead calmed the mind and gave clarity of thought, while Ibn Sina, the famous Arabian philosopher of the tenth century, compared its powers to that of a magnet. To the Rosicrucians, jacinth symbolizes the true knowledge of absolute love. In the eighteenth and nineteenth centuries, colorless zircon was called Matara diamond.

Some writers connect zircon with the signs of Leo, Virgo, and Sagittarius.

To dream of a deep orange or red zircon signifies success after a stormy period. Dreams of green zircon symbolizes incoming money, while colorless and light blue mean spiritual growth.

▶ **HEALING ENERGIES:** Helpful with liver diseases and loss of appetite.
Brown or brownish red: heals headaches.
Red: ear infections.

▶ **MAGICAL POWERS:** A stone of quiet vibrations, zircon enables one to be at peace with oneself. A stone of great purity, zircon can create unity with the Higher Self and spirit guides.
Brown: grounding.
Colorless: clears the aura; severs cordings.

Colorless and yellow: clears the entire aura, brings sleep, and gives wisdom in stressful times. Attracts love.

Green: helps one open up to make new friends; draws in wealth.

Light blue: balances, uplifts, stabilizes the mind and emotions.

Pink: helps with astral travel at night during sleep.

Red: heals injuries and soothes pains.

Violet: draws money.

MAGICAL USES

Zircon is a versatile stone that works well in any ritual, spell-working, meditation, or as a divination aid. It can be substituted for many more expensive stones without much loss of energy and power.

Part III

Other Uses For Stone Magic

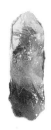

Practical Spell-Magic with Stones

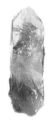

There is no end to the number of various ways to use stones and crystals in rituals and spellworkings. You need to be very familiar with the vibrations and energies emanating from each of your stones so you will intuitively know how they should or should not be used in magic. The following magical workings are a few examples of how I have been led, through the instructions of my spiritual teachers, to use stones.

SOUND AND CRYSTALS

The use of sound through crystal points is an ancient art that is just now being rediscovered. Although this procedure does not require any advanced magical skills, it does require patience, practice, and persistence. You can also do this by yourself, as no helper is required, unless you wish or you need your own chakras cleared. This method can be used to intensify healings, ease pain, or empower candles and other objects that will be used in spellworkings. If you are proficient in magical working already, you can use this method in combination with visualization of a desired goal to increase the speed with which it manifests.

You do not have to search for a special toning or singing crystal to use this magical application. All you need is a small C tuning fork and a crystal point of clear quartz, amethyst, smoky quartz, or citrine. Clear quartz can be used for any procedure; smoky quartz works best against pain or disease caused by something in a past life or in the past of this life. Amethyst and citrine are best for cleansing chakras and opening blockages.

The crystal *must* have a point that is not damaged. At no time should you ever strike the crystal with the tuning fork. The fork is only held near the base of the crystal once it has been struck.

If you plan to do healing or ease pain, hold the crystal point downward over the site of disease or pain. Strike the tuning fork lightly against a firm object, and then hold it close to the base of the crystal. The sound runs down through the crystal point into the damaged area, thus changing the body vibrations into a more positive tone. This may take several applications before the result is felt. Never use the toned crystal more than twice on one spot at a session.

If you want to cleanse and unblock your chakras using a crystal and sound, you will need someone you trust to work on you. Lie flat on your back and relax. The person with the tuning fork and crystal point should start at the root chakra and work up to the crown chakra. Hold the crystal above each chakra in turn and strike the tuning fork. Hold the fork near the crystal and leave it there until the vibration completely stops. Repeat with each chakra up to and including the crown of the head. Never tone a crystal twice on a chakra at a session, as the vibrational change will be too extreme and may make the patient feel nervous or ill.

If charging candles or other objects for magical use, perform this method within a cast circle. Hold the crystal over the object and strike the tuning fork. Close your eyes and visualize what energy you want to penetrate the candle. Do this two more times to reinforce the energy entering the candle or object. Leave the empowered objects on your altar overnight.

STONE HEALING WITH POPPETS

To many people, the use of a poppet brings up a negative mental image of pins and black magic. However, poppets are used far more frequently to heal than to hurt. If you are a visual person (one who understands things better if you see them), you should be able to use this method without any problems. This method can be used for healing whether or not you know what the disease is or can pinpoint an exact spot.

A poppet is a small cloth doll in the rough shape of a human and with eyes, nose, and mouth marked. It is usually lightly stuffed with cotton and can be purchased in various colors. If you have any sewing skills, you can make your own without problems. The best colors of poppets used in healing are blue, pink, or green. The best time to do this healing is at least two days after a New Moon.

For this stone method you will need a poppet, pen, small knife, and seven small crystal points. The crystals can be either clear or amethyst; smoky quartz is not advisable for this method. Write the name of the person needing the healing directly onto the poppet, or onto a small paper that you can then pin to the doll. Make seven tiny incisions in the poppet at the site of the seven chakras. Insert a crystal into each incision, beginning at the root chakra and ending at the crown chakra. All the points of these crystals should be pointing upward out of the doll.

Hold your hands over the poppet and say: "*The negative energy flows out, to be released and reformed. Only positive energy flows in, to heal and balance.*" As you take a breath, visualize the positive energy flowing down into the crystals; as you exhale, see the dark negative energy flowing up out of the crystals.

Put the poppet where it will not be disturbed. Repeat the chant once a day for seven days.

CHAKRA ALIGNMENT WITH STONES

Sometimes you will need to be more specific on a healing than just using clear crystal points. Other times you might simply want to work on realigning your, or someone else's, chakras gently over a period of time. If you have a typical household, one with pets and/or children who are curious about stones, you need to have a more secure setting than the top of your altar or sacred space, especially since you will want to leave this method working for weeks, perhaps longer.

You will need a shoebox (or similar) with a lid, paper and pen, and a small piece each of the following stones: 1) garnet, black obsidian, or smoky quartz; 2) carnelian; 3) tiger's-eye or citrine; 4) green jade, aventurine, rose quartz, or watermelon tourmaline; 5) azurite or lapis lazuli; 6) sodalite, sugilite, amethyst, purple fluorite, or clear quartz; 7) amethyst, clear quartz, or blue, white, or gold fluorite.

Outline the shape of the box's bottom on a sheet of paper. Draw a rough human shape onto the paper with an X marking each of the chakras. Write the name of the person the picture represents below the feet in the drawing. Cut out and lay this paper into the box.

As you set the appropriate stones in place on each X-marked chakra point, chant: "*The power flows and spirals strong, the wheels turn with strength and might. The energy path is pure and clear, as it reaches to new heights.*"

Run your hand above the stones, from the root to the crown chakra, three times, or until you feel the energy flowing in that direction. Put the lid on the box and leave in a place where it will not be disturbed for seven, eleven, or twenty-two days. Once every seven days, repeat the chant.

STONE PENDULUMS AND WANDS

Wands and pendulums are common items in any Pagan's supply of spellworking tools. Usually, one wand and one pendulum are used for all purposes, and this does work well for most things. However, there comes a time when a magician wants to experiment with something new. Different stones do work best for different magical divinations and/or rituals, although having a different wand or pendulum for each procedure is not absolutely necessary to the working of magic.

Rather than go to the time and expense of looking for ready-made wands and pendulums of the correct stones, you can make your own with only a little effort. The stones need not be very large; in fact, it is better if they are not. Large stones make the wand top-heavy and difficult to use. Such stones in pendulums make it more difficult for the astral energies to move. Larger stones do not necessarily mean more power, either.

To make your own wands, you can use short, sturdy pieces of dowel, not more than twelve to sixteen inches long. Although a long wand may seem more impressive, the length makes it awkward in spellworkings.

to the bedroom. If the crystal point does not have a bail, see above how to wrap it with silver wire.

Hang the crystal point over the head of the bed by a piece of blue thread. Put the turquoise, moonstone, or tiger's-eye on the left side, the onyx on the right, and the obsidian at the foot. If necessary, attach them to the mattress as described above. Burn a small amount of rose or lotus incense in the room.

If your dreams become too intense, or you feel as if you have been studying all night, you might have to remove the stones for a week or so.

GEODE CAVE

There are times in everyone's life when the need to pull back and regroup energies in preparation for the beginning of another cycle of events is felt. This can occur because of an actual life cycle, or it can be used to stimulate the beginning of another cycle. Changes can be frightening, hard on the energies and nerves, especially if those in the past have been negative experiences. To avoid the negativity engendered by the uncertain beginning of a cycle, you can "retreat" into a geode cave of rebirth to help you gain control of both yourself and the situation.

Several hundred dollars for a two-foot-high geode is out of the question for most people. Size is not so important as is the way you feel about a certain geode. Since you will be traveling mentally and astrally into the geode cave, a small geode will work just fine.

When you have chosen your geode and taken it home, spend time just looking at the fantastic arrangement of the crystal inside it. Hold the geode in both hands and listen to the intuitive feelings and impressions you receive. Become familiar with it, until you can imagine it as a huge natural cave into which you could walk.

When you are ready to enter this magical realm, close your eyes and visualize yourself going into the "cave." Explore this crystal-lined paradise in short reverie or in a deeper meditation. Feel the pulsing waves of energy from the crystals, almost like a heartbeat. Do this until you feel at peace and safe in the geode cave.

If you are struggling with a life cycle, now is the time to draw energy and wisdom from the crystals to help you. Touch the crystal-lined walls; embrace the larger stones. Tell the stones what you need to handle the cycle with positive vibrations, and listen to the thoughts they send back to you. Little by little, you will find small changes occurring in the cycle, enabling you to move closer to the goals you set. This technique will also work if you are trying to end one cycle and begin another one. Often after spending time in the geode cave, you feel as if you were reborn.

If you are pregnant, or about to share becoming a parent, you can enter the geode cave and ask to contact the spirit of the unborn child. The crystals will help you make contact and bond with this new spirit. This method will also expose the child at a very early age to the power of crystals, possibly reawakening psychic abilities from other lifetimes.

CRYSTALS AND LIGHT

Quartz crystals and colored lights have been used for years in healing. Here is a method for using them together to speed up healing and/or chakra cleansing.

You will need a clear quartz crystal large enough to hold easily, a small penlight or flashlight, and small colored pieces of photographer's lens material. This colored plastic can be purchased in sheets in photography or hobby stores. Cut a piece of each color and tape it with clear tape over the lighted end of the flashlight as needed.

For healing, the colors blue, pink, and green are the most effective. Hold the crystal, point toward the diseased area, and shine the colored light through the crystal. Hold it there no longer than one minute at a session. In cases such as fevers, use a blue light over the spleen, to cool and balance. The pink color is a gentle healer, especially for small children; red is too harsh for most people and tends to aggravate "hot" or inflamed conditions. Green is very good for nervous conditions, where agitation has resulted from the illness itself or from traumatic events.

When working on the chakras, match the color to the appropriate chakra. Follow the color work with just the white flashlight in a quick sweep from the root to the crown centers. Always begin chakra work on the lowest, or root, chakra, and end at the crown.

You can also use this colored-light method to intensify the power in candles, spell-bags, or wish-papers before you burn them on your altar.

Red: root chakra; Muladhara.[1] Survival, grounding, courage to face a conflict or test, taking action, energy. Use in healing when the patient is suffering from great loss of energy and has no inflammation of any kind.

Orange: belly chakra; Svadhisthana. Changes, possible moves, changing your luck, control of a situation, sexuality. Use for those who have blood problems, problems with sexuality or the sex organs, or rheumatism.

Yellow: solar plexus chakra; Manipura. School, study, creativity, mental pursuits, sudden changes. In healing, use for those who have digestive problems.

Green: heart chakra; Anahata. Prosperity, career, jobs, marriage, long-term relationships, creativity, balance. Useful in healing for heart trouble, flu, colds, tension headaches.

Blue: throat chakra; Visuddha. Good health, recovery from illness, harmony, understanding, journeys. Respiratory illnesses, throat troubles, and blood pressure respond well to this color.

Indigo: third eye or brow chakra; Ajna. Development of psychic abilities, discovering past lives, seeing and handling karmic problems, stopping undesirable events. Use for insomnia, depression, or sinus problems.

Violet or lavender: crown chakra; Sahasrara. Spiritual growth, breaking bad luck, success in long-range plans, protection. This color works well on anxiety, migraines, some insomnia, and intense pain that has lasted some time.

The following colors are of value to chakra healing but have no specific connection with any particular chakra.

Pink: friendships, children, pets, true love. Pink helps in healing deep grief, loneliness, and insecurity.

Brown: contact with Nature spirits, common sense, success.

White: general life pattern, spiritual guidance, being centered, seeing past illusions, guidance into the right paths.

STONE STAR WEBS

Each of the following stone star webs is illustrated to help you lay out the stones in the proper places. It helps if you draw or trace the design out on a sheet of paper and then place the stones. This makes it easier to trace the connecting lines with the forefinger of your power hand, the final step after placing the stones. This physical action must be done to set each spell in action and activate the powers flowing through the web. You should make the last connection by ending up where you started in tracing the design. Except for the twelve-point star, all star webs are activated by tracing in a clockwise direction. These star webs can be left in place as long as you want; just retrace the energy paths once a day.

Celtic Triangle: This three-point design helps with communicating with the Triple Goddess and represents the balance of manifested desires. It also can be used for creativity, pregnancy, and children. Set a single-terminated amethyst crystal at the top angle, a lapis lazuli on the lower left, and a green or watermelon tourmaline on the lower right. Begin the activation by tracing from the top point to the lower left, then to the right angle.

Four-Point Star: I prefer this design of a four-point star rather than the typical cross. To me a cross represents suffering and torture, not the energies a magician wants to activate in positive magic. This diagram symbolizes the Four Elements: Earth, Air, Fire, and Water. It is also used in learning to work with the Elements, create balance and completion, and bring in stability. It helps in communicating with the God. Put a single-terminated smoky quartz at the top angle. A piece of red jasper is placed on the left angle, blue agate or shell on the right, and a small meteorite or tektite at the bottom. Begin the tracing at the smoky quartz and move clockwise.

Five-Point Star: This design is also known as a pentagram in pagan and Wiccan circles. It represents the magician's control of earth energies and her/his reaching toward the spiritual. It is used for gaining spiritual insight into physical problems. Place a piece of amazonite at the lower left angle, then amber at the top point. Put pyrite at the lower right angle, fluorite at the left crosspiece, and aventurine at the right crosspiece. Begin the tracing at the lower left where you placed the amazonite and follow each line just as you placed the stones.

Seven-Point Star: Traditionally, this star design is thought to be a symbol of perfection and seven has long been considered to be the most sacred of all numbers; it was also the Egyptian symbol of life eternal. To modern magicians, the seven-point star represents the Goddess, the God, and Nature combined in humans. Known as the mystic star, this design is excellent for contact and study with astral spiritual teachers and guides. Begin at the upper left angle and put a piece of lapis lazuli there. Moving clockwise along the lines of the design put the following stones at the proper point, in the order in which they are given here: carnelian, obsidian, malachite, moonstone, tiger's-eye, and meteorite or tektite. Activate the power paths by tracing the lines just as you put down the stones.

Eight-Point Star: This web design is good for regeneration; strength and growth after traumatic events; switching life into a new cycle; spiritual advancement by correcting and balancing karma; or balancing your physical and astral forces and energies. Beginning at the upper left angle, and moving clockwise, place the following stones in the order given: garnet, clear quartz, green tourmaline, amethyst, Boji stones, aventurine, galena, and moss agate. Trace the power lines in the same direction.

Nine-Point Star: A traditional symbol of spiritual initiation, this star web can be used to gain prophetic and guiding dreams; bringing things to an end and preparing for a new cycle; or for finding and understanding mystical wisdom.

This web pattern actually consists of three triangles; the power of three tripled; the Triple Goddess multiplied three times. The first triangle symbolizes the spiritual; the second, the astral; the third, the physical. Begin the first triangle at the upper left angle with a clear quartz crystal; moving clockwise, place next an emerald, then an amethyst. The second triangle begins at the upper right angle and moves clockwise; start with lapis lazuli, then jade or serpentine, and finally blue topaz. The third angle begins at the right-hand angle, just below the starting point of the second triangle. Here, place a red agate, followed by watermelon tourmaline and bloodstone. To activate, trace each triangle in the same pattern in which you laid out the stones, always moving clockwise. Begin with the spiritual triangle, and end with the physical one.

 Ten-Point Star: This star web design is very useful in magic for or about your career; properly activated, it symbolizes satisfactory completion. Start at the upper left angle with a carnelian; moving clockwise, lay out the other following stones: lapis lazuli, bloodstone, clear quartz, obsidian, galena, tiger's-eye, red jasper, moss agate, and amber. Activate by tracing along the lines in a clockwise direction from the first stone.

 Twelve-Point Star: The twelve-point star is actually a representation of the zodiac, or the manifested universe. Each point symbolizes a house of the zodiac. Use this star web whenever you feel your entire life is out of balance. It is also useful when you are going through a difficult time caused by disturbing progressed aspects to your natal chart.

Zodiac houses: 1) personality, tendencies, outlook; 2) financial affairs, material possessions; 3) relatives, siblings, studies, mental abilities; 4) home, environment, the God, father, domestic affairs; 5) children, love affairs, speculations; 6) work, health, small animals; 7) marriage, partnerships, lawsuits, contracts, open enemies; 8) legacies, taxes, death, astral experiences; 9) long journeys, foreign countries, dreams, visions, psychic experiences, education, intuition, spiritual tendencies; 10) career, profession, public life, honor, fame, the Goddess, mother, employer; 11) friends, hopes and wishes, associations, society; 12) unexpected troubles, limitations, secret sorrows, self-undoing, secret enemies, large animals, the occult.

Place the following stones at the correctly numbered point of the diagram and moving counterclockwise. 1) Boji stones; 2) lodestone; 3) sard; 4) clear quartz; 5) aventurine; 6) carnelian; 7) fossil;

8) moonstone; 9) jade; 10) smoky quartz; 11) staurolite; 12) amethyst. To activate the power paths, trace the design counterclockwise from the starting point.

LIGHTNING ZIGZAG

Sometimes you need a series of energy bursts to break down hindering barriers to reaching your goals. The Lightning Zigzag is excellent for this use. You will need a small clear crystal cluster and a piece each of lodestone, lapis lazuli, tiger's-eye, moss agate, and a single-terminated amethyst crystal. This is one stone layout that works best if the pattern is actually marked out in some way. You can draw it on paper or use strips of masking tape or flat ribbon. See the illustration.

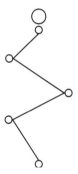

Begin by laying the first stone at the top of the zigzag and finish with the last stone at the bottom. When all the stones are in place, you can activate this energy pattern by placing the forefinger of your power hand against the base of the amethyst and simply saying: "Begin!"

The Zigzag is a lightning, or running pyramid, pattern—a path and pattern of specific stones that intensifies the flowing energy each time it ricochets from one stone to the next. The amethyst point draws energy out of the astral, adds this to its own power, and sends it racing down the path. At the end, the lodestone pulls all the energy together and feeds it into the crystal cluster in pulsating bursts, like repeated lightning strikes.

The crystal cluster sits at the end of the zigzag; write out your desired result on a small piece of paper, fold it, and tuck it into the cluster. Place the lodestone so that it touches the crystal cluster. Next out is the lapis lazuli, followed by the tiger's-eye and moss agate. Place the single-terminated amethyst crystal at the other end of the zigzag, with the point directed at the moss agate.

I suggest that you "shut off" the energy before dismantling the Zigzag. Do this by placing the forefinger of your power hand against the base of the amethyst and saying: "Stop!"

I set up a Zigzag, using thin copper wire to mark the path. A curious visitor picked up the tiger's-eye out of the pattern without permission and got a physical shock from the pulses of disrupted energy. She shortly developed a severe headache and upset stomach. Although her manners about snooping around have not improved, she no longer picks up any of my stones, and her visits are now infrequent.

TANGLING WEB

This stone pattern works well if you need to stop someone's interfering with any part of your life. This can be on the physical, astral, or magical levels. It literally entangles the person's psychic energy and makes it virtually impossible for her/him to continue causing you problems. See the illustration.

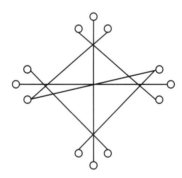

This is another pattern that works best when the web path is drawn out on paper or marked out with masking tape or flat ribbon. If you know the perpetrator's name, write it on a small piece of paper and place the paper in the center of the web. Place the eight pieces of onyx or obsidian in their proper places, then the four pieces of hematite. As soon as the last stone is set in place, the Tangling Web begins to operate.

NEGATIVE GIVING AND RECEIVING PATTERN

Before anyone panics, this is not how to send negativity to someone else. This method of spellworking with stones is to prevent certain auric vampires in human form from siphoning off your energy. You know the kind: people who show up tired out and pessimistic and who leave pumped up and cheerful, while you feel drained. This will also work to deflect negative thoughtforms or deliberately sent negative energy coming from others who are jealous, angry, or just plain out to make trouble for you. Of course, this will not work as well if you are living with the vampiric person in question.

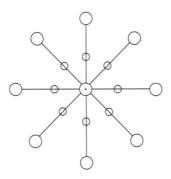

To operate as a negative giving pattern, this stone layout should be placed on an altar or in some sacred space where it will not be disturbed until you choose to dismantle it. The pattern is based on the eight-spoke Celtic wheel design. In the center set a clear quartz crystal; this will be the psychic generator that will coordinate the power of the other stones. The inner row should be eight pieces of onyx or obsidian, set in the exact pattern in the diagram. The outer row should be of single-terminated amethyst or smoky quartz crystal points; all the points should be aimed inward. When the pattern is completely set up, touch the center crystal with your power hand and say simply: "You are activated."

It is best to set up this stone pattern after the New Moon. Each day, carefully touch the center crystal to be certain you are connected with its protective power. It can be left in place as long as you wish.

If you are dealing with deliberate psychic, astral, and/or magical attack, you can set out the same pattern, but on a larger scale, on the floor, as a negative receiving pattern. The only difference is that the single-terminated crystals should all point outward, not inward. After setting the outer two rows of stones in place, sit in the middle and hold the center crystal in both hands. This places you within the psychic protective field of the stones, both physically and astrally. When you feel it is safe to leave, and you have soaked up enough stone power to feel secure, simply place the central crystal in its proper place and step out of the pattern. This will have forged a strong link between you and the stones, a connection that will stay in place for several hours. Most people who dabble in dark magic do not have the skill or patience to keep at it steadily for any length of time. However, the ones dedicated to the dark side do have great skill and patience, so you should be prepared to perform this ritual again if necessary.

MYSTIC SPIRAL MANDALA

The Mystic Spiral Mandala, with its thirteen stones, is a spiritual energy pattern to strengthen and transform you, as a person. Before using this pattern, however, be very certain you actually want the deep-reaching changes that will come. Prepare yourself mentally and spiritually for the transformation, as it can be a rough experience. Fully understand that such transformations will affect every part of your life.

The center is a shooting star, clear quartz pointed crystal; second is the Moon, moonstone; third is the Egyptian ankh, carnelian; fourth is the Chinese longevity symbol, beryl; fifth is the butterfly, galena or meteorite; sixth is the Nordic wealth symbol, garnet or green zircon; seventh is the Celtic trefoil, malachite; eighth is the Greek owl of wisdom, fluorite; ninth is crossed swords, hematite; tenth is flowers, moss agate, or holey stone; eleventh is stylized waves, fossil, or shell; twelfth is a mountain, aventurine; thirteenth is a dragon, lapis lazuli.

Each of the pictures symbolizes a specific goal needed in life. The shooting star: successfully reaching your goal. Moon: psychic development. Ankh: spirituality. Longevity: health. Butterfly: family, friends. Wealth: prosperity, success. Trefoil: balance. Owl: wisdom, knowledge, study. Crossed swords: action, protection. Flowers: happiness. Waves: travel, moves, changes. Mountain: career. Dragon: catalyst to change.

The web power path is activated by tracing inward from the dragon to the shooting star. The energy movement is also from the position of the dragon inward, in a continuing spiral until it reaches the shooting star in the center. From there, the accumulated energy is released in bursts as it builds.

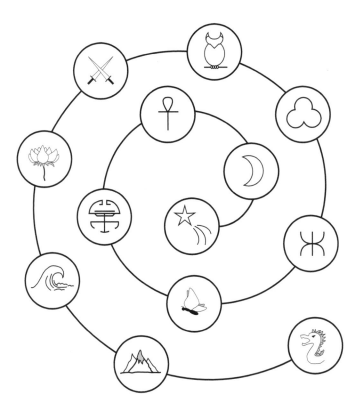

RINGS FOR THE FINGERS

You can wear rings containing certain stones to bring about magical changes in your life. You might choose certain stone-rings because you will be facing a particular set of circumstances today. Or you might choose rings that will affect certain areas of your life that need help every day. Last, but not least, you might wear certain stones to counteract difficult aspects in your natal chart. Choose the stone in a ring according to what you wish to accomplish. Then to double the action, wear that stone on a specific finger.

The art of palmistry has long associated each finger of a hand with a particular planet. Using the following definition list of the thumb and fingers, you can decide how to wear your rings.

Thumb—will power, logic, temperament, physical vitality.

Forefinger—Jupiter; ambition, success, relationships, marriage.

Middle finger—Saturn; karma, fate, philosophy or religion, study.

Ring finger—Sun (Apollo); personality, happiness, artistic talents, career.

Little finger—Mercury; creativity, communications, the psychic, intuition.

Stone Bead Crafts

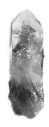

Many rock shops and lapidary shows now offer beads made from various stones for sale. These stone beads can be used in a variety of ways, simply because certain colors or types please the eye of the craftsperson or for their specific spiritual and magical qualities. Anyone already involved in beading can easily adapt these pierced stones to their craft. For those new to beading, I have included a few simple projects that are decorative, meaningful, and fun.

DREAM CATCHERS

Dream catchers have become very popular today through a resurgence of Native American culture. Although such dream catchers on the market look much like a spider's web, there is no reason that one cannot be made in another design. Pagans may wish to use the pentacle (five-point star) or the ancient Sun symbol, two of their symbols. After all, the purpose of this implement is to snare nightmares, and any woven design will do this.

Some children and adults are particularly frightened by bad dreams. It is difficult to rationalize such fright or explain it away. One of the best methods of helping the person to cope is to hang a dream catcher above the head of the bed. Dream catchers do work. They are symbols of personal control over dreams. And the subconscious mind that creates dreams only understands symbols.

A pentacle dream catcher is not difficult to make. It requires a circular ring, small beads, and some thread, string, crochet thread, or small gauge wire to weave the design upon this ring. If you use wire, you may also find it necessary to use a small pair of pliers to tighten the wire around the ring. You also need to decide whether you want each crossing strand of thread or wire to be filled with beads or whether you want only a few token beads on each strand.

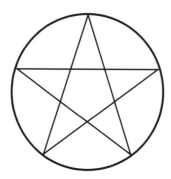

For beads on both the pentacle and Sun dream catchers you might choose agate (healing), amber (change), amethyst (pleasant dreams), beryl (prevents psychic manipulation), fluorite (enhances the powers of other stones), garnet (prevents bad dreams), red jasper (prevents magical attack), lapis lazuli (reduces tension), malachite (helps with sleep), onyx (repels negative energy), quartz crystal (balances emotions), tiger's-eye (grounding), or turquoise (aligns the chakras). If you are striving for a more aesthetically pleasing look, you may decide to use only certain colors or colors that compliment each other, rather than dwell on the magical meanings.

To begin, tie or fasten one end of the thread or wire to the ring. Measure the thread to the opposite side of the ring, put on the beads you desire, and then wind the thread around the opposite side of the ring three times at a slight angle from the original attachment, pulling it tight. This will be part of the left leg of the pentacle. Each time you attach the thread to the ring, wind it three times.

Now attach more beads and wind the thread about the ring a short distance from the first tying. Your design should look like an inverted V-shape. Put on more beads and pull the thread to the left side of the ring, winding it about the ring a little more than half-way up the side. Adjust it until it looks like the lower angle of the cross-arm of the pentacle. Thread the beads and stretch the string to the opposite side, winding it about the ring. For the finishing angle, again put on the beads and pull the thread back to the point of beginning.

If you carefully check the angle of the thread each time you prepare to wind it at another point on the ring, you can adjust the design. Make a small loop for hanging at the top of the pentacle. If you wish to further decorate the ring, cut three equal pieces of thread or wire. Thread the beads on each string, anchoring the first bead by bringing the thread or wire through the bead and up, tying it near the entry point. Then thread on the other beads. Tie each thread to the bottom of the pentacle ring an equal distance apart. This provides a nice movable decoration.

For the Sun dream catcher you will need a larger ring and a much smaller ring for the center, thread or wire, and beads. Attach the thread to the top center of the larger ring. Put on the beads, then wind the thread around the top center of the small ring. Continue the string and beads through the center of the smaller ring and wind it about the bottom center of the smaller ring. Continue with the beads and string and attach to the bottom center of the larger ring. By careful adjustment of the stringing thread, you can situate the smaller ring in the exact center of the larger one. Knot and cut the thread.

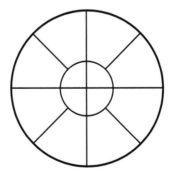

Attach the thread to the left center of the larger ring, thread on the beads, and wind about the left center of the smaller ring. Continue with the thread and beads through the small ring and attach to the right center of the larger ring. You now should have a decoration that looks like a cross within a large circle with a smaller circle in the center. Knot and cut the thread.

To finish, tie a bead-strung thread between each of the threads on the outer, larger ring and attach them to the smaller ring. Knot and tie off each string. Do not run these on through the center. When you are finished, the design will resemble the Celtic eight-spoke wheel with a smaller, crossed ring in the center.

Let your creativity flow, and you will find that a number of different possibilities for dream catchers will present themselves.

OTHER BEAD GIFTS AND CRAFTS

Let your imagination soar when working with stone beads. You can make jewelry for yourself or others that is unique and inexpensive. The presently popular metal neck-ring can be enhanced by attaching a large bead or a series of beads. Bracelets can be made by stringing beads on jewelry or copper wire; just be sure to make it big enough to easily slip over the hand. Stone beads can be added to key chains, hair laces, or threaded onto small wire and attached to earrings. Making your own gifts using stone beads allows you to personalize the gift according to the person's needs. Stone gifts may be given for birthdays, weddings, anniversaries, graduations, absolutely any occasion that you might want to celebrate.

Many people worry that combining different stones will have a negative or nullifying effect of the energies, as if there are right and wrong combinations. I have not found this to be true. The Goddess and God were quite ingenious when They created the powers within stones. These powers work together perfectly and in harmony, with the only exception being the occasional stone that does not feel "right" to a specific person.

If you wish to tailor a gift very specifically for your own or another person's individual needs, read back through the previous section on stones and make a list of those that are primarily for the purpose you have in mind. Just use common sense, and remember to substitute less expensive stones for those that are out of reach in price. Having a true alexandrite or star sapphire, for example, might mentally sound nice, but it is not using common sense to purchase a stone that costs more than you make in a year or two. Everyone has necessary priorities in life, and having such an exorbitantly priced stone should not be one of them.

Have fun with stones and stone beads. Even if you do not consider yourself to be a creative person, give it a try. It is a relaxing, easy pastime that you can enjoy without being a world-class creator of jewelry. I have a small stone with black felt glued on the bottom to resemble a turtle's appendages. It was a gift made years ago by one of my children. You never know what a simple gift, made by hand with love, will mean to someone else.

Stone Divination

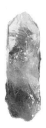

Foretelling the future by divination has been around almost as long as humans have lived upon the Earth. A number of different methods have been used: runes, stones, pendulum, shells, the behavior of animals and birds, scrying, and cards. One of the most common practices, and easy to learn how to do, is divination by stones. In European countries, the method of casting lots, runes, or stones became known as sortilege, a word that comes from the French words *sorcier* ("male witch") and *sorciere* ("female witch").

There are two simple methods of casting and reading stones: one where each stone represents a planet or specific activity; the other where each stone has its own special meaning.

For planetary stone divination, get thirteen stones: ten for the astrological planets, plus one each for magic, life, and home. Choose one each of the stones from the following list of suggestions. The stones are chosen primarily for color, not necessarily for the magical meaning.

Choose one each out of each following category. Sun: gold tiger's-eye, pyrite, goldstone. Moon: cloudy white quartz, moonstone, white chalcedony. Mercury: hematite, galena, labradorite. Venus: rose quartz, coral, malachite. Mars: bloodstone, red jasper, garnet. Jupiter: lapis lazuli, blue topaz, amethyst. Saturn: black onyx, obsidian, black tourmaline. Uranus: Iceland Spar, flint, picture jasper. Neptune: pearl, shell, blue-green tourmaline. Pluto: petrified wood, tiny geode, tektite. Magic: small ammonite, holey stone. Life: carnelian. Home: moss agate.

Keep your divination stones in a small soft bag and cast them onto a dark-colored cloth. Black and dark blue are traditional colors that show the colored stones to their best advantage. However, you could also use a piece of white velvet for the same effect. Frame your question clearly while holding the stones. Then toss them gently onto the cloth. The stones are read according to the general pattern in which they fall. If two or more stones lie close together, that is a center of power that is important; closely aligned stones also influence each other's power.

The Sun stone represents a good influence, God, or masculine influences. The Moon is feminine influences, Goddess, journeys, and psychic things. Mars portends struggle, problems, confrontations, and possible danger. Mercury is for news or messages, writing, travel, study, and communications of all kinds from verbal and books to television and films. Jupiter means good luck, money, job, and opportunities. Venus symbolizes love, friendships, and artistic things. Saturn stands for restrictions, karma, or troubles out of the past. Uranus means unexpected changes, possible arguments or altercations, and having to deal with things you have put off in the past. Neptune has to do with religion or spirituality (growth, changes, or problems), psychic experiences, or creative ideas. Pluto symbolizes the end of one cycle and the beginning of another, death and rebirth, or a startling inner transformation (positive or negative).

The life stone is simply the life and health of the person asking the question, while the home stone signifies personal property, real estate, or the actual dwelling in which you live. The magic stone represents the power of the deities or that generated by rituals and spellworkings, as well as the unexpected serendipitous events of life.

For a simple yes or no question, use the magic stone and the Sun and Saturn stones. If the Sun stone is closest to the magic stone, the answer to your question is yes. If the Saturn stone is closest, then the answer is no. If the Sun and Saturn stones are of an equal distance to the magic stone, then the outcome is doubtful, scrambled, or not jelled enough yet to predict.

For another method of foretelling with stones, use the following stones and their definitions. You can have more than one of each type of stone if you wish. Draw out the illustration onto a cloth and embroider it, use colored cloth paint, or just mark it in black lines.

Gently roll the stones in the bag until they are well mixed. Concentrate on the question you want answered. Without looking, reach into the bag, choose a stone, and lay it on the cloth to the East. The next stone is placed in the South, the next West, the next North, and the last in the center.

The East stands for ideas, thoughts, inspiration, psychic abilities. The South is for action, passion, change, perception of situations. The West represents emotions, healing, marriage or relationships, love. The North is the region of prosperity, money, growth, success, business or employment. The center of the cloth stands for the power you are using, either negative or positive, to affect the question.

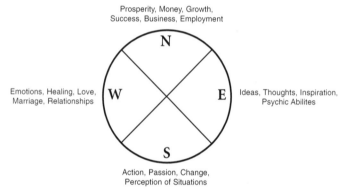

Read each stone according to the direction in which it lies, then in relation to the other stones. For example, if black onyx is in the South, it points to present events or situations that have their roots in the past; some change you want or perception you have is influenced by karma. Lodestone in the West would indicate coming good fortune in relationships, while clear quartz in the East shows intuitive guidance that will help you make the right decisions. Amazonite in the North indicates news coming about employment or finances. If hematite, for example, is the center stone, which influences all the other stones on the cloth, it signifies that if you take action and responsibility you can get a favorable outcome to the question.

You can use this layout to determine whether a proposed action will prove beneficial to you, or whether you should re-think your plans. You may need to make minor changes for a better outcome, or possibly scrap the idea altogether.

STONE MEANINGS

Amazonite: news or messages will soon be arriving.

Amber: finances will improve; a new source for prosperity will open.

Ammonite: intuition and dreams will be important in reaching a decision.

Aventurine: good luck is coming.

Black Onyx: the present problem or dilemma has roots in a past life or in the past of the present life. Deal with it this time and get rid of the karmic ties.

Bloodstone: you need to see through an illusion that is impeding your progress. This can be from yourself or another person.

Carnelian: a possible change or improvement in career. Strengthens any stones that fall into the same quarter with it.

Clear Quartz: your intuition will guide you to the correct answer to things that are puzzling or bothering you.

Cowrie Shell: a possible pregnancy or period of great creative productivity.

Fluorite: you will be studying or learning something new that could be vital to your future.

Green Jade: you need to let go of strong, old emotions.

Green Tourmaline: an unpleasant experience will turn out to be good luck for you.

Hematite: favorable outcome to a problem if you take action and accept responsibility.

Holey Stone: an illness will soon be resolved.

Lapis Lazuli: important dreams or psychic experiences will help you out of a rut.

Lodestone: money, love, or good fortune in general can be yours with a little effort.

Malachite: a journey is in the near future.

Petrified wood: a stagnant situation is about to break loose.

Pyrite: a relationship problem with a friend or co-worker will ease.

Red Jasper: be alert. There are those around you who might cause harm by word or deed if they think they can get away with it.

Rhodonite: a period of stress.

Rose Quartz: a new love or friendship is near.

Rhodonite: a period of stress.

Sard: a pleasant family gathering.

Tektite: you have allowed yourself to get too tired. Relax and get back your energy.

Tiger's-Eye: the truth you have been seeking will be revealed.

Scrying with Stones and Stone Mirrors

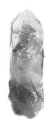

People who are interested in divination eventually want to try divining or scrying with a crystal ball. The crystal ball has long been a traditional tool for gazing into the future, and fascinates us with its mystery and messages. What most people do not realize is that the ball or sphere is not the only way to look into the past, present, or future. There are other simple tools that work in the same manner.

The practice of scrying is known around the world, in nearly every ancient culture. The word *scry* comes from the word *descry*, which means to reveal. The word is used to describe the magical art of gazing into a stone globe, a polished, flat slab (mirror), or a vessel of water for prophecy and visions. The scrying device has also been called a speculum. Although the word speculum came to mean a magical mirror or ball during the Middle Ages, there have been other devices used with just as much success. Many of the ancient references to special chalices, such as "Jamsheed's seven-ringed-cup" in the *Rubaiyat of Omar Khayyam*, are descriptions of scrying devices. Traditions worldwide speak of people using pools of water, special wells, puddles of ink, chalices of wine, or shimmering jewels.

The practice of crystal gazing may be as old as fifteen to eighteen thousand years. Archaeologists have found crystal spheres in such places as Siberia, Australia, Chaldea, Greece, Rome, Assyria, Persia, Japan, China, France, Ireland, and Scotland. In the Yucatan Peninsula of Mexico, the ancient Mayan and Aztec foreseers used a clear stone they called *zaztum*; they not only used spheres but egg-shaped stones as well.

The monks in Tibet knew crystal balls as "the windows of the gods" and treated them as holy objects with great powers. Buddhist altars often held crystal spheres, believing them to symbolize emptiness.

Most of our present information on scrying comes from ancient manuscripts. Various methods of scrying are well documented in surviving literature as far back as the Greek and Roman times. Before this time, we can only rely on archaeological finds and ancient wall paintings.

Pausanius, a Greek writer, told of a method in the Temple of Demeter (Ceres) at Patras. The temple had a special well with steps that led down close to the water. The scryer would lower a mirror on a cord so that it just barely touched the water. The visions were seen in the reflection on the mirror. Crystal balls have been recovered from ancient tombs and funerary urns throughout the Mediterranean and Middle East.

An ancient Orphic poem, entitled "*Lithica*," tells of a black magical sphere used for divination. The substance of which this ball was made was called *sideritis* or *ophitis*; no one has an accurate translation of these words, although we feel certain the stone referred to is the present day siderite. During the Trojan War, a male soothsayer named Helenus used a heavy, dark globe of siderite to correctly predict the downfall of the city. Helenus treated this globe as a living being and made offerings to it until it developed the distinct personality of a living soul.[2]

Siderite, which comes in shades of brown, from very pale to very dark, has long been considered as a magical stone. Chalybite is another name for siderite; this name comes from the Greek and Roman word for iron or steel, a term that arose from the Chalybes, an early tribe of Asia Minor who were noted ironworkers. Iridescent siderite, a unique form of this stone, is found in Bisbee, Arizona.

However, scrying goes back much further than the Greeks and Romans. In ancient Mexico, tradition says that the Aztec god Tezcatlipoco had a magical black mirror in which he could see everything that happened in the world. Flat polished mirrors of black obsidian or onyx have been found among the temple ruins of that culture, a clue that at least the priests engaged in divination using this method. Obsidian and clear quartz crystal were treated as valuable divination tools; copal incense was burned before them as an offering. Later, Apache medicine men of the southwestern United States used ordinary crystals to induce visions and find lost property.

Although pagan practices were under attack during medieval and later times, scrying was often condoned. The practice of ceremonial magic, which was church-oriented in its use of deity names, was frequently performed, and basically went unpersecuted by the church if the practitioners were male. Many of the clergy and priests were known to have engaged in ceremonial magic. In one sixteenth-century manuscript the writer tells of a certain scrying crystal even being placed on the church alter. A manuscript written in 1658 by a Capuchin priest describes an "earth-mirror," or *Erdenspiegel*, which seems to be nothing more than a magical mirror.

During the medieval times, it was widely believed that the magician trapped a spirit inside the stone or mirror through powerful magic, and that this spirit had no choice but to give visions and predictions. It was a common practice for the wealthy to employ a household scryer, just as they would have a private physician or servants.

The famous Dr. John Dee of England first used a crystal ball on December 22, 1581. Eventually, Dee owned more than one scrying device. Besides the crystal ball, he had a ball of cairngorm and a polished slab of black obsidian. Only his scrying ball of Scottish cairngorm (smoky quartz) is today in the British Museum. Dee used a red silk cloth under the scrying devices instead of the usual black ones. He was a prominent figure of his time, an astrologer as well as a prophet, and was popular with both Queen Elizabeth I and the Emperor Rudolph II.

As the orthodox church amassed more and more power, however, even ceremonial magic came under attack. During the days of witch persecutions and the burning times, the church and witch-hunters believed that every scrying stone held a demon, imprisoned there through magical practices that somehow included their devil. If anyone prophesied using such a device, then she/he was consorting with evil spirits, which by law was a capital offense punishable by death. Since the church controlled secular laws as well as church laws, the art of scrying had to be practiced in strict secrecy.

Card reading and the practice of the religion of Wicca eventually came under the same disfavor as scrying. The ruling church pressured the governments of many countries to pass laws against these practices. Although secular governments felt confident enough to fight against the old church-dictated death sentence, they bowed to the idea that such behavior was wicked and needed punishing. An English law, passed in 1824, sent crystal readers to prison for three months' hard labor as rogues and vagabonds. This and similar laws were not repealed until the mid-1900s.

Divination by scrying was practiced during medieval times in other countries besides those of Europe. Ibn Kaldoun of Persia (b. 1332) wrote about crystal gazing. Another Arabian author, Haly Abou Gefar, wrote of a golden ball used by the Magi, who followed the Zoroastrian religion. This sphere was set with a sapphire and attached to a strip of bullhide. To divine, the magician watched the golden ball while swinging it rapidly in a circle. This idea was probably taken from the much earlier Goddess religions in Crete and Greece where a similar sphere was used for prophecy.

Globes of crystal, beryl, onyx, and obsidian have been used as scrying stones for thousands of years. So have flat polished pieces of these stones. They have been called scrying, seeing, or show stones. Until recent times, when laws against Wicca or witchcraft were rescinded, many Pagans used dark-colored fishing floats or silver-coated ornaments as scrying balls to avoid persecution by church and authorities. Others would drop a silver coin into a black cauldron filled with water.

Today, the most popular and common scrying device is a clear crystal ball. Large pieces of natural clear crystal, relatively free from inclusions, are nearly impossible to find, and upon finding them are exorbitantly expensive. It is extremely difficult and outrageously expensive to purchase a sphere of natural crystal of any size. Any sphere over an inch in diameter is very rare and priced far above what the majority of people would pay. Most clear crystal quartz is too flawed to produce spheres of any size. Only two large natural crystal balls have been produced within the last 100 years; one crystal came from Madagascar and was 6 1/8 inches in diameter, the other from Calaveras County in California was 5 1/2 inches.

Manmade crystal is more frequently used as crystal balls. These show stones are set in a pedestal of wood, glass, or metal to prevent their rolling around. Some globes or balls will have a small flat section that enables them to sit firmly.

If you wish to try your hand at scrying, do not spend a lot of money on a crystal ball in the beginning. Size is only to impress others. A large size and high price do not indicate power in either a sphere or stone of any shape.

In the beginning, it is best to choose a smaller sphere of crystal or any stone that appeals to you. In the opaque spheres, a dark color, such as black or very dark brown, seems to work best. For example, black obsidian, even with gold, silver, or rainbow sheen, makes an excellent scrying sphere. Even though they might not be perfectly round, the obsidian balls fashioned in Mexico are of excellent quality. If you can find a rainbow obsidian with an eye, you truly have a treasure. Remember, bigger does not mean better or more powerful. Each sphere or mirror must be judged on its own.

If you decide to work with a "mirror," a flat, polished slab of black onyx or black or deep brown obsidian is the best to use. Slabs can be more difficult to find, as they are not as flashy and as connected in the public's mind with scrying as is the sphere or ball. However, they can be just as powerful as the sphere and will cost much less.

To scry, all one needs is a polished surface of some kind. This can be a crystal, onyx, beryl, or obsidian ball; a flat polished slab of stone; the surface of water; a pool of ink; or even a globule of quicksilver. Even one flat side of a clear crystal point will work.

The basics of scrying are actually quite simple. The person gazes into the shiny surface with half-closed eyes until the optical nerve gets tired and ceases to report what it physically sees. The scrying device seems to disappear from sight and a mist gathers in its place. The subconscious mind can then send up pictures, symbols, or mental impressions. Scrying visions appear to fall into two categories: symbolic visions, which must be interpreted, and the clear pictures of events. Scrying should not be done for more than a few minutes at a time, as fatigue will block the psychic abilities.

Before using any scrying stone or mirror, you should cleanse it and then consecrate it with incense. One method of cleansing a globe or mirror is to hold it under cool running water for a few minutes. Another method is to imagine that its surface is turning black, and that every vibration within the stone is being sucked up by the blackness and removed. After washing the stone carefully in cool water, dry and wrap it in a dark cloth, such as black, green, purple, or blue. The Full Moon is an excellent time to charge the scrying stone.

Traditionally, a dark-colored cloth such as black, blue, green, or deep purple is placed underneath the globe or mirror to create a non-reflective background. Such materials as silk, velveteen, or velvet work nicely.

When using the globe or mirror, sit with it at a comfortable level before you. No light—electric, sun, or candle—should reflect directly into it while you first begin working. At a later time, you might find that candlelight is not distracting, but helpful. Some pagans believe that the scrying ball or mirror works best only after sunset. I have not found this to be totally accurate, but I prefer to scry in at least a semi-darkened room. Pass your hands several times above and around the ball to magnetize it; the right hand should move clockwise, the left counterclockwise. Look into the ball, adjusting your point of vision deep into the surface. Relax; blink if necessary. Work no longer than ten minutes in the beginning. Some writers recommend working with the scrying stone within a consecrated circle.

Do not try to analyze anything that happens, just flow with it. Soon you will feel as if you are being pulled into the globe or mirror. You may feel as if you are shrinking and that you are separated from your body. The first few tries should be merely getting acquainted with the feel of your scrying stone. When you are comfortable, ask a specific question before you begin gazing.

With whatever kind or shape of stone you use for scrying, be certain that you ask a very clear question before using it. Or ask the crystal to show you either the past, the present, or the future as it applies to your life. The scrying stone can open you to psychic information in many ways and help in meditation.

Rather than staring at the surface of your scrying stone, instead look deep within it. Allow yourself to relax and drift into a borderland state between the physical and the astral. This opens your inner mind to psychic influences. Be patient, though, as it may take a lot of practice for this to happen. When you cease to be aware of the scrying stone, the thoughts and mental pictures will appear. The first signs of visions may be clouds or streamers of mist, sometimes only white, other times in various colors. Be very careful that you do not interpret the pictures and symbols as you want your answer to be.

Patience, practice, and perseverance are the key words in learning how to scry. Keeping a journal of your progress and what you see is also helpful. Record everything, even though you think it is of no importance. You must discover how your subconscious mind feeds you information.

Colored or white mists floating in one direction may indicate something positive, while if they float in the opposite direction, it may be a negative sign. Certain colors may have specific meanings to you. Giving a list of color meanings is not always helpful, as one person may interpret red, for example, as one thing, while to a second person this color would have a totally different meaning.

The same applies to symbols. To cat lovers, a cat means love, freedom, and connection with the psychic, while dog lovers would not respond favorably to those meanings at all. Although some symbols have retained the same meanings for thousands of years, others are open to individual interpretation, or at least to shadings of interpretations. That is why dream books are ninety percent useless. Symbols are personal communications with your own subconscious mind and the superconscious, or universal race mind, described by Carl Jung.

Perhaps the most important suggestion for scrying, whatever the device you decide to use, is to do it for fun and not to try too hard. As with the development of any psychic ability, if you push too hard and long your subconscious mind gets tired and frustrated. It will stop cooperating. The only person you need to impress is yourself, just as the only person you have to prove anything to is yourself.

If you still have difficulties "seeing" things in the mirror or sphere, try closing your eyes and looking for pictures inside your head while holding your scrying device. You may well discover that you see colored pictures clearly in your mind. Or you may begin getting clear psychic feelings and impressions that are just as accurate as the pictures others see within their device. Never measure yourself against the way others scry or what they see.

Even if all of these methods do not seem to open the astral doors into your scrying device, you do not need to give up. Use the stone as a dream enhancer by placing it under your pillow or beside your bed. Hold it during meditations to strengthen your psychic connections with your teachers and guides. No stone is ever worthless, if you just take the time to work with it.

Stone Patterns for Healing

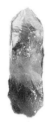

The use of stones in healing is a very ancient practice that is coming back into use today. As with all types of metaphysical, alternative healing, please use this method in conjunction with standard medical treatment, not just by itself.

All healing with stones should not be longer than fifteen minutes at any one session. When first working these stone patterns on a new patient, be aware of the patient's body language of comfort or discomfort while the stones are in place. Some people are unable to tolerate the stones for even as long as five minutes in the beginning.

At no time should you ever tape stones directly to the body and leave for any length of time! This can cause an imbalance in itself, creating even greater problems.

Have the patient dress in comfortable clothing and lay flat on her/his back. Do the healing in a calm, quiet place where you will not be interrupted. Playing soft instrumental background music will help the patient relax. Take your time and do not rush.

First, arrange the stones required on the appropriate places on the body. Then position the larger clear quartz crystals. Activate the outer quartz crystals by tapping each one gently in the pattern sequence explained in the description of each stone pattern. These crystals will automatically activate at your touch and energize the stones situated on the body. After each healing, take care to wash all used stones and crystals thoroughly under cool running water.

STRESS RELIEVER

Most, if not all, disease is brought about by a weakening of the body and its natural defenses in some manner through stress. To begin healing, stress must be greatly reduced or eliminated. Sometimes stress has become such a part of the life pattern that a boost of some kind is needed to get the patient headed in the right direction. The stone pattern called Stress Reliever is an excellent place to begin, as well as a gentle way to introduce a patient to stone healing.

Stones required for the Stress Reliever pattern are: three large clear quartz crystal points; an amethyst for the brow; two small amethyst points, one for the palm of each hand; two smoky quartz crystals to be placed near the soles of the feet; and a piece of rose quartz and a small clear crystal point (point upward) to be placed on the abdomen near the navel.

Ask the patient to close his/her eyes and concentrate only on the music and the visual image of floating comfortably on a fluffy cloud, a calm lake, or a big bed. You might wish to discuss which you will suggest by talking to the patient before the healing. Some people have a great fear of heights or water and will not be comfortable if you use those suggestions. Assure them that at no time will they have the sense of falling, but will remain calm and comfortable. Gently position the body stones first, followed by the outer crystal points.

The Stress Reliever sets up two separate triangle areas of energy. The top triangle begins at the crystal above the head, descends to the crystal near the patient's left hand, crosses to the crystal by the right hand, and ascends to join the crystal at the head. Activate the stones in this triangle first by following this sequence.

The lower triangle consists of the rose quartz and small crystal point on the abdomen, descends to the smoky quartz by the left foot, crosses to the smoky quartz by the right foot, and ascends to join the rose quartz. Activate the stones in this triangle in this sequence.

When the healing is finished, you need to deactivate the quartz crystals before you remove the stones or allow the patient to get up. Do this by gently tapping each outer quartz crystal or stone gently in the exact pattern sequence you used to activate them.

When the patient first arises, have him/her sit quietly for a few moments to avoid dizziness, headache, or disorientation.

CHAKRA CLEANSING

Everyone gets their seven chakras out of balance, polluted, or partially closed merely from trying to live in this modern, high-paced life. This stone pattern will gently open, realign, cleanse, and balance the energy flowing through the chakras, thus not only healing, but making life a little easier to handle every day.

Stones required for the Chakra Cleansing pattern are: four large clear quartz crystals for the outer pattern; a small clear quartz point to be set near the crown of the head; amethyst for the brow; lapis lazuli for the throat; rose quartz for the heart; tiger's-eye for the abdomen; carnelian for the spleen area; garnet for the root (or genital) area; a small crystal point for the palm of each hand; and smoky quartz to be placed near the sole of each foot.

Ask the patient to close her/his eyes and concentrate only on the music and the visual image of floating comfortably on a fluffy cloud, a calm lake, or a big bed. Again, you might wish to discuss which you will suggest by talking to the patient before the healing. Some people have a great fear of heights or water and will not be comfortable if you use those suggestions. Assure them that at no time will they have the sense of falling, but will remain calm and comfortable. Gently position the body stones first, followed by the outer crystal points.

The outer pattern of clear quartz crystals here forms a double triangle, or two triangles set base to base. Activate this crystal energy flow by tapping the large crystal at the head, down to the one by the left hand, descend to the crystal at the feet, up to the one by the right hand, and ascend to join the crystal at the head again.

When the healing is finished, you need to deactivate the quartz crystals before you remove the stones or allow the patient to get up. Do this by gently tapping each outer quartz crystal gently in the exact pattern sequence you used to activate them.

When the patient first arises, have him/her sit quietly for a few moments to avoid dizziness, headache, or disorientation.

PAST-LIFE CLEANSING

This stone pattern is often necessary when everything else seems not to work well. It really does not matter if the present problems arose from the past of this life or past lives of other times. Each of us carries hundreds of old tapes in our subconscious mind, tapes of events and/or habit patterns that can surface in this life to create havoc and disease without our willing them to do so.

Some patients will find themselves watching or reliving old experiences or old lives without warning. Be alert to any sign of distress or discomfort, ending the healing session quickly if necessary.

This stone pattern is to release any lingering effects of any type of past life. The patient needs to release, so that healing can take place, whatever the root cause of the problem. After the patient is lying down, instruct her/him to immediately release any negative emotions or remembrances as soon as they come into her/his mind. One way to do this is for the patient to see her/himself dropping the negative images into a well.

Stones required for the Past-Life Cleansing pattern are: five large, clear quartz crystals for the outer pattern; lapis lazuli for the brow; turquoise for the throat; tourmaline (either pink or watermelon) for the heart; rose quartz for the abdomen; amber for the palm of each hand; and black obsidian to be placed near the soles of the feet.

Ask the patient to close her/his eyes and concentrate only on the music and the visual image of floating comfortably on a fluffy cloud, a calm lake, or a big bed. You might wish to discuss which you will suggest by talking to the patient before the healing. Some people have a great fear of heights or water and will not be comfortable if you use those suggestions. Assure them that at no time will they have the sense of falling, but will remain calm and comfortable. Gently position the body stones first, followed by the outer crystal points.

The outer pattern of quartz crystals is activated in the form of a five-point star. Begin by tapping the crystal near the patient's right foot, then the one over the head, down to the left foot, up to the crystal near the right hand, across to the one by the left hand, and back to the crystal at the right foot.

When the healing is finished, you need to deactivate the quartz crystals before you remove the stones or allow the patient to get up. Do this by gently tapping each outer quartz crystal gently in the exact pattern sequence you used to activate them.

When the patient first arises, have her/him sit quietly for a few moments to avoid dizziness, headache, or disorientation.

Personal Gemstones

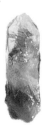

Although wearing zodiacal gems was practiced for centuries in ancient cultures, particularly in the Middle and Far East, this practice was not popular in Europe until about 1500 C.E. The practice of wearing birthstones may go back as far as 6,000 years. A Egyptian High Priest's tomb (dated at 4,000 B.C.E.) yielded a breastplate with twelve different stones. Now certain gems are also associated with various anniversaries as well.

The following lists vary from source to source. It is seldom that any two lists are identical. I believe it is up to the individual to select which stone feels proper to her/him as a birthstone. If you are familiar with your natal chart, you may decide to wear or use stones which represent your ascendant (rising sign), Moon sign, or a sign in which you have a number of influencing planets. Or you may determine that you need to select stones corresponding with planets whose influence you need; these you can wear for certain periods of time to create magical changes in your life.

STONES OF THE SEASONS

Spring	Summer	Autumn	Winter
peridot	ruby	golden topaz	moonstone
amethyst	fire opal	sapphire	rock crystal
pink topaz	pyrope garnet	smoky quartz	turquoise
morganite	uvarovite garnet	tourmaline	labradorite

GEMSTONES OF THE ZODIAC

Aquarius	Jan. 20–Feb. 18	garnet/turquoise/hawk's-eye
Pisces	Feb. 19–March 20	amethyst
Aries	March 21–April 20	red jasper/bloodstone/carnelian
Taurus	April 21–May 20	rose quartz/carnelian/sapphire
Gemini	May 21–June 20	citrine/tiger's-eye/agate
Cancer	June 21–July 20	emerald/chrysoprase/aventurine
Leo	July 21–Aug. 21	rock crystal/onyx/citrine
Virgo	Aug. 22–Sept. 22	yellow agate/carnelian/citrine
Libra	Sept. 23–Oct. 22	smoky quartz/citrine/peridot
Scorpio	Oct. 23–Nov. 22	red carnelian/aquamarine/sard
Sagittarius	Nov. 23–Dec. 20	chalcedony/topaz
Capricorn	Dec. 21–Jan. 19	ruby/onyx/cat's-eye

GEMS FOR THE BIRTH MONTH

January	rose quartz/garnet
February	amethyst/onyx
March	red jasper/bloodstone/aquamarine
April	white sapphire/diamond/clear quartz
May	emerald/agate/chrysoprase
June	moonstone/pearl
July	onyx/turquoise/ruby
August	peridot/aventurine/sardonyx
September	chrysolite/sapphire/lapis lazuli
October	opal/beryl/tourmaline
November	topaz/tiger's-eye
December	ruby/zircon/turquoise

STONES FOR THE WEEKDAYS

Monday	pearl, moonstone
Tuesday	ruby
Wednesday	sapphire
Thursday	garnet
Friday	emerald
Saturday	diamond
Sunday	topaz

STONES FOR THE THIRTEEN MOON MONTHS

The Moon months, and the dates given for each month, come from my book *Moon Magic*. The thirteenth month is arbitrarily only a few days long, a dating system widely used by the Celtic cultures.

1. Wolf Moon—January—labradorite, moldavite, or selenite.
2. Ice Moon—February—clear crystal, diamond, or sugilite.
3. Storm Moon—March—amethyst, coral, or hiddenite.
4. Growing Moon—April—chrysocolla, chrysoprase, or jade.
5. Hare Moon—May—emerald, peridot, or green zircon.
6. Mead Moon—June—amber, malachite, or pearl.
7. Hay Moon—July—ruby, garnet, Padparadscha, or Mexican fire opal.
8. Corn Moon—August—Boji stones, carnelian, or quartz cat's-eye.
9. Harvest Moon—September—cinnabar, opal, or pyrite.
10. Blood Moon—October—flint, red jasper, or spinel.
11. Blue Moon—October 27–November 1—obsidian, spectrolite, jet, or moonstone.
12. Snow Moon—November—galena, hematite, or sodalite.
13. Cold Moon—December—lapis lazuli, uvarovite, or petrified wood.

WEDDING ANNIVERSARIES

Many cultures in Asia and the Far East consult the local astrologer before embarking on any major undertaking, especially marriage. The astrologer works out the best day and time for the marriage. Then he will suggest the best gem to be worn on certain anniversaries, how long to wear it, and whether the stone should be set in such a way in jewelry that it touches the skin.

I have chosen gemstones to replace the other materials often associated with wedding anniversaries, so this list is not entirely traditional.

1. amber	17. amethyst
2. carnelian	18. garnet
3. pearl	19. zircon
4. onyx	20. emerald
5. malachite	23. sapphire
6. amethyst	25. silver
7. turquoise	30. pearl
8. jade	35. coral
9. peridot	40. ruby
10. lapis lazuli	45. alexandrite
11. copper	50. gold
12. agate	52. star ruby
13. moonstone	55. emerald
14. moss agate	60. diamond
15. rock crystal	65. star sapphire, gray
16. topaz	67. star sapphire, purple

BUDDHIST SEVEN PRECIOUS MINERALS

1. gold	5. cat's-eye
2. silver	6. diamond
3. pearl	7. coral
4. sapphire or ruby	

HINDU STONES OF THE DIRECTIONS

Center	Sun	ruby
East	Venus	diamond
Southeast	Moon	pearl
South	Mars	coral
Southwest	North Node	jacinth (zircon)
West	Saturn	sapphire
Northeast	Jupiter	topaz
North	South Node	cat's-eye
Northwest	Mercury	emerald

These stones were often set into a talisman, known as the "nine-gem" jewel.

STONES OF THE MOSLEM SEVEN HEAVENS

1. emerald
2. white silver
3. large white pearls
4. ruby
5. red gold
6. jacinth
7. pure shining light

CHAKRA STONES

1. garnet, black obsidian, smoky quartz.
2. carnelian, Mexican fire opal.
3. tiger's-eye, citrine.
4. green jade, aventurine, rose quartz, watermelon tourmaline.
5. azurite, lapis lazuli.
6. sodalite, sugilite, amethyst, purple fluorite, clear quartz.
7. amethyst, clear quartz; blue, white, or gold fluorite.

STONES FOR PSYCHIC SENSE DEVELOPMENT

1. Seeing	emerald, beryl, aquamarine, obsidian
2. Touch	carnelian, smoky quartz
3. Hearing	onyx, amber
4. Smell	jasper, agate
5. Taste	topaz, tourmaline

ANGELS, PLANETS, DAYS, SEASONS, AND STONES

Angels	Planet	Day	Season	Stone
Aniel/Anael	Venus	Friday		emerald
Attarib			Winter	moonstone
Camael	Mars	Tuesday		lodestone
Cassiel		Saturday		jet
Gabriel	Moon	Monday		clear crystal
Haniel	Venus	Friday		holey stone
Kafziel	Saturn			tektite
Khamael or Zamael		Tuesday		fire agate
Michael	Mercury	Sunday		goldstone
Raphael	Sun	Wednesday		agate
Sachiel	Thursday			lapis lazuli
Sammael	Mars			bloodstone
Spugliguel			Spring	peridot
Torquaret			Autumn	topaz
Tubiel			Summer	garnet
Uriel, Auriel	Mars			ruby
Zaphiel, Orifiel	Saturn			onyx

ANGELS, MONTHS, ZODIAC SIGNS, AND STONES

Angel	Month	Zodiac	Stone
Adnachiel	November	Sagittarius	azurite
Ambriel	May	Gemini	geode
Asmodel	April	Taurus	moss agate
Barbiel	October	Scorpio	citrine
Barchiel	February	Pisces	beryl
Gabriel or Cambiel	January	Aquarius	iolite
Hamaliel	August	Virgo	amazonite
Hanael	December	Capricorn	fluorite
Machidiel	March	Aries	aventurine
Muriel	June	Cancer	Iceland Spar
Uriel	September	Libra	ametrine
Verchiel	July	Leo	heliodor

STONES FOR THE TWELVE PLANETS OF ASTROLOGY

Sun: yellowish or gold-colored stones, such as amber, hyacinth, topaz. (Chaldean, diamond). Planetary attributes: money, health, prosperity, publicity, success, fame, rank and high office, hope.

Moon: whitish stones, such as moonstone, diamond, crystal, opal, beryl, mother-of-pearl. (Chaldean, selenite, or moonstone). Planetary attributes: intuition, women's affairs, motherhood, visions, public contact, emotions, water.

Mars: reddish stones, such as ruby, hematite, jasper, bloodstone. (Chaldean, ruby). Planetary attributes: military, policemen, fire fighters, bravery, destruction, justice, strength, war, sexual energy, surgery, power over enemies.

Mercury: neutral tinted stones, such as agate, carnelian, chalcedony, sardonyx. (Chaldean, agate). Planetary attributes: writing, publishing, messages, teaching, travel, bookkeeping, secretarial work, speaking.

Jupiter: bluish stones, such as amethyst, turquoise, sapphire, jasper, blue diamond. (Chaldean, jacinth). Planetary attributes: riches, honors, employers, law, judges, bankers, foreign affairs, career success, speculation.

Venus: greenish stones, such as emerald, some sapphire, some zircon. (Chaldean, emerald). Planetary attributes: love, friendships, the arts, pleasure, appearance, children.

Saturn: black stones, such as jet, onyx, obsidian, black coral, black tourmaline, black diamond. (Chaldean, sapphire). Planetary attributes: wills, legacies, old age, property, mines, the deceased, karma.

Uranus: blue-green stones, such as turquoise, malachite, amazonite. Planetary attributes: sudden changes, transformation, inventive thought, new ideas.

Neptune: lilac and violet stones, such as amethyst, opal. Planetary attributes: imagination, artistic sensitivity, religion (as opposed to spirituality), the mystic, drugs, addictions.

Pluto: dark red stones, such as dark red agate, pryope garnet, almandine garnet. Planetary attributes: death and rebirth, mysteries, beginnings and endings, hidden problems.

Asteroids (called Lucifer by some): mother-of-pearl stones, such as opal, moonstone, and certain shells.

Earth: brown stones, such as leopard agate, fire agate, titanite, staurolite, Vesuvianite, cassiterite, and smoky quartz.

OTHER NAMES FOR CERTAIN STONES

Achroite	See Tourmaline.
Almandine	See Garnet.
Andradite	See Garnet.
Apache Tears	See Volcanic Glass.
Balas Ruby	See Spinel.
Bone Turquoise	See Fossils.
Brazilian Topaz	See Citrine.
Cairngorm	See Smoky Quartz.
Carbuncle	See Ruby and Garnet, Almandine.
Cat's-Eye	See Alexandrite, Crocidolite, and Cat's-Eye
Cinnamon Stone	See Garnet.
Copralite	See Fossils.
Cross Stone	See Staurolite.
Cymophane	See Cat's-Eye.
Demantoid	See Garnet.
Desert Rose	See Barite.
Dravite	See Tourmaline.
Eye-Stone	See Agate, Cat's-Eye, Crocidolite, Tiger's-Eye, Hawk's-Eye.
Fairy Cross	See Staurolite.
Gaggitis	See Jet.
Galaktite	See Jet.
Grossular	See Garnet.
Heliotrope	See Bloodstone.
Hessonite	See Garnet.
Hyacinth	See Zircon.
Iceland Spar	See Calcite.
Indicolite	See Tourmaline.
Jacinth	See Zircon.
Jargoon	See Zircon.

Magnetite	See Lodestone.
Marcasite	See Pyrite.
Melanite	See Garnet.
Morion	See Smoky Quartz.
Mother-of-Emerald	See Plasma.
Mother-of-Pearl	See Shell.
Mount Saint Helen's Stone	See Volcanic Glass.
Nephrite	See Jade.
Obsidian	See Volcanic Glass.
Olivine	See Peridot.
Phantom Quartz	See Quartz.
Pyrope	See Garnet.
Quartz Cat's-Eye	See Crocidolite.
Rhodolite	See Garnet.
Rose Quartz	See Quartz.
Rubellite	See Tourmaline.
Rutillated Quartz	See Quartz.
Sardine Stone	See Sard.
Schorl	See Tourmaline.
Scottish Topaz	See Smoky Quartz.
Smoky Quartz	See Quartz.
Soapstone	See Steatite.
Spectrolite	See Labradorite.
Spessartine	See Garnet.
Tektites	See Meteorite.
Topazolite	See Garnet.
Tourmalinate Quartz	See Quartz.
Tsavolite	See Garnet.
Vesuvianite	See Volcanic Glass.
Zoisite	See Tanzanite, Thulite.

GLOSSARY OF TECHNICAL TERMS

Allochromatic: gems colored by impurities; without these, the gem would be colorless.

Asterism: the star effect seen on some gems when they are cut *en cabochon*.

Cabochon or *en cabochon*: a special cut given to a gem; this is a domed upper surface that helps to create chatoyancy, asterism, or displays the gem and its color to better advantage.

Carat: the standard unit of weight used internationally to measure gems; 0.2 grams.

Chatoyancy: the cat's-eye effect seen in certain types of stones when cut *en cabochon*. When the gem is turned and the light plays across it, a thin line of light gives the same effect as an eye.

Cleavage: lines of weakness within a gem where the gem-cutter can break the stone in order to show it at its best advantage.

Cryptocrystalline: the mineral structure where the crystals are too small to be seen even with a microscope.

Crystal systems: the way crystals are grouped according to symmetry. There are six main systems: cubic, monoclinic, triclinic, trigonal/hexagonal, orthorhombic, and tetragonal.

Dendritic habit: branching, or tree-like formations.

Dichroic: two colors; the color effect in certain gemstones; when turned one direction in the light, one specific color is seen; when turned another, a different color appears.

Double refraction: a gem's ability, because of its structure, to bend light, so that any image seen through the transparent stone has two images.

Doublet: a manufactured stone made of two pieces of mineral or substance glued together.

Facet: the cut and polished surfaces of a gemstone.

Fire: the splitting of white light into the rainbow colors of the color spectrum.

Fluorescence: an optical effect where a mineral appears a different color under ultraviolet light.

Geode: a cavity inside a rock, with crystals lining its inner surface, all growing toward the center.

Heat treatment: application of heat to a gemstone to enhance or change its color or clarity.

Imitation gemstone: a manmade gem; does not have the physical properties of the gem it imitates.

Inclusions: foreign bodies or markings within a stone. Crystals of one mineral that are encased within another.

Intergrowth: two or more crystals that are attached to each other.

Iridescence: the effect of light reflecting off internal features of a stone; this produces rainbow-like colors or flashes. Sometimes this looks like a film of oil on water.

Luster: the shine of light off a stone's surface.

Massive: minerals that have an indefinite shape, or small crystals in masses.

Matrix: the parent or host rock in which a gem is found.

Meteorite: a rock that comes from outer space, through the atmosphere to the Earth.

Microcrystalline: a mineral whose crystals are so small they cannot be seen without a microscope.

Moh's scale of hardness: measurement of a stone's hardness in relation to other minerals. The scale devised by the Austrian mineralogist Friedrich Mohs.

Multicolored: single crystals composed of different colored parts.

Opalescence: a milky blue form of iridescence.

Organic gem: a gem derived from living organisms.

Paste: glass made to look like real gems.

Piezoelectric/piezoelectricity: the generation of positive and negative charges in a stone when pressure is applied.

Pleochroic/pleochroism: a gem that shows two or more colors when viewed from different angles.

Polycrystalline: a mineral composed of many small crystals.

Prismatic crystal: a crystal that is longer in one direction than in the other.

Refraction: the bending of light as it passes through a crystal.

Rough: a rock or crystal in its natural state.

Schiller or sheen: a form of iridescence.

Specific gravity: the density of a mineral or gem compared with an equal amount of water.

Synthetic: a laboratory-made gem whose chemical composition and optical properties are very similar or identical to the natural stone.

Translucent: a stone that allows light through it, but cannot be clearly seen through.

Transparent: a stone that allows light through and also can be clearly seen through.

Triochroic: a gem that shows three different colors or shades of color when viewed from different directions.

Twinned crystals: two or more crystals of the same mineral that grow together in some manner.

Volcanic bomb: a blob of lava thrown out of a volcanic and which solidifies before it hits the ground.

STONE QUALITIES AND POWERS

Not all of each stone's influences, qualities, and powers are listed here. Before using a stone for the description listed, read the text on that particular stone for appropriate color and type.

Abuse, surviving: iolite, jasper, kunzite, lapis lazuli, smoky quartz, rhodocrosite, spinel, tourmaline, obsidian.

Accidents, preventing: carnelian, chalcedony, malachite, turquoise, spinel, topaz.

Actors: quartz, scapolite, tourmaline.

Adjusting: quartz.

Adventures: aventurine, cinnabar.

Alertness: agate, jet.

Align bodies: amazonite, carnelian, emerald, lodestone, marble, peridot, quartz, rhodocrosite, tourmaline.

Ancestors: quartz.

Anger: chrysocolla, jade, marble, peridot, rhodonite, ruby, serpentine, topaz.

Artists: aventurine, emerald, quartz, tourmaline.

Astral travel: moss agate, carnelian, galena, lodestone, meteorite, petrified wood, quartz, sapphire, shell, zircon.

Aura: moss agate, Boji stones, citrine, fluorite, ivory, jet, spectrolite, lapis lazuli, opal, quartz, topaz, tourmaline, obsidian, zircon.

Authorities, government: bloodstone.

Bad habits: agate, amazonite, citrine, obsidian.

Balance: agate, amethyst, aquamarine, aventurine, calcite, carnelian, chrysoprase, emerald, ivory, jade, kunzite, spectrolite, lepidolite, lodestone, malachite, moldavite, moonstone, onyx, opal, quartz, rhodocrosite, serpentine, sodalite, sugilite, tanzanite, thulite, tiger's-eye, topaz, tourmaline, turquoise, vanadinite, obsidian.

Beauty: alabaster, chalcedony.

Bleeding, controlling: bloodstone, jasper.

Blockages, removing: aventurine, calcite, jasper, kunzite, malachite, quartz, rhodocrosite, ruby, sapphire, shell, sodalite, obsidian.

Burglars, deterring: topaz.

Business: amethyst, citrine, garnet, jade, malachite, marble, opal, quartz, sard, serpentine, spinel, tourmaline, obsidian.

Calming: adularia, agate, amber, amethyst, aquamarine, aventurine, chrysoprase, coral, fossils, ivory, jade, kunzite, lapis lazuli, lepidolite, marble, onyx, peridot, quartz, rhodocrosite, rhodonite, serpentine, sodalite, tanzanite, topaz, tourmaline, zircon.

Caregivers: quartz, titanite.

Centering: amber, aventurine, galena, quartz.

Chakras: agate, amber, amethyst, aventurine, fluorite, ivory, jasper, lapis lazuli, lodestone, malachite, opal, quartz, rhodocrosite, tourmaline, turquoise.

Changes: amethyst, peridot, quartz, smoky quartz, obsidian.

Change vibrations: agate, quartz.

Channeling: amethyst, fluorite, quartz, sapphire, sugilite, obsidian.

Children: coral, lapis lazuli, quartz.

Cleansing: azurite, lapis lazuli, opal, peridot, quartz, selenite.

Combining: ametrine, fossils, spinel.

Communications: agate, amazonite, aventurine, beryl, chrysocolla, garnet, lapis lazuli, malachite, moldavite, sodalite, spinel, tourmaline, turquoise.

Concentration: carnelian, fluorite, quartz, spinel, topaz, tourmaline.

Conflicts: agate, tourmaline.

Consciousness-altering: quartz.

Control: garnet, hawk's-eye, jet, onyx, sapphire, thulite.

Courage: agate, diamond, hematite, jade, ruby, serpentine.

Court cases, lawyers, the law: amethyst, aquamarine, chalcedony, hematite, jade, lodestone, sard, serpentine.

Creativity: agate, amazonite, amethyst, apatite, aquamarine, aventurine, chrysocolla, chrysoprase, emerald, jade, lapis lazuli, malachite, onyx, opal, quartz, sapphire, serpentine, sodalite, spinel, topaz, tourmaline, turquoise, obsidian.

Cycles in life: tiger's-eye, obsidian.

Dark magic, defeating: amethyst, holey stones, mica, onyx, peridot, petrified wood, pyrite, quartz, sapphire, sard, topaz, tourmaline, obsidian.

Deceptions: moonstone.

Deflects negativity: beryl, jasper, quartz.

Demonic possession, removing: jet.

Destiny: peridot, quartz.

Diagnosis: quartz.

Discrimination: agate, spinel.

Divination: agate, amethyst, hawk's-eye, cat's-eye, crocidolite, moonstone, quartz, rhodocrosite, tiger's-eye, tourmaline. See Psychic abilities.

Dreams: agate, amethyst, emerald, jade, quartz, rhodocrosite, serpentine.

Dream stone: garnet, jade, quartz.

Earth energy: aventurine, smoky quartz, staurolite, wulfenite.

Earth spirits: quartz, staurolite, wulfenite. See Nature spirits.

Education: see Teachers.

Elements, Four: fossils, quartz, staurolite, wulfenite.

Empathic: aventurine, goshenite, heliodor, quartz.

End of the rope: malachite.

Enemies, defeating: aquamarine.

Energy: agate, andalusite, beryl, goldstone, jasper, quartz, rhodocrosite, rhodonite.

Energy shield: tektite, rhodocrosite, tourmaline.

Evil spirits, repelling: agate, bloodstone, carnelian, crocidolite, jade, jasper, malachite, onyx, serpentine, tourmaline, obsidian.

Excessive energy, removing: fluorite.

Extraterrestrial energies, contacting: meteorite, tektite, quartz, topaz, tourmaline.

Fairies: see Nature spirits.

Family problems: carnelian, sard.

Fear: amber, aquamarine, aventurine, chrysocolla, citrine, coral, fossils, tourmaline, obsidian.

Feminine energies: chrysocolla, jade, moonstone, turquoise.

Fertility: See Pregnancy, Creativity.

Fire, protecting against: topaz.

Friends: agate, geode, iolite, lapis lazuli, ruby, sard, topaz, tourmaline, turquoise, zircon.

Gambling: aventurine, lodestone.

God: amethyst, ammonite, quartz.

Goddess: amethyst, ammonite, jet, moonstone, quartz, shell.

Good luck: agate, amethyst, aventurine, carnelian, holey stones, lodestone, onyx, opal, petrified wood, sapphire, sard, staurolite, tiger's-eye, topaz.

Grief: tourmaline, obsidian.

Grounding: agate, fluorite, smoky quartz, serpentine, tiger's-eye, obsidian, zircon.

Guardian angels: quartz.

Guilt: chrysocolla, tourmaline.

Hallucinations, controlling: jasper.

Happiness: moss agate, amazonite, amethyst, garnet, marble, ruby, sapphire, sard, zircon.

Harmonizing: aventurine, calcite, coral, jade, lapis lazuli, lepidolite, quartz, serpentine, sodalite, obsidian.

Headaches, treating: aventurine, hematite, jet, lodestone, turquoise.

Higher Self: citrine, diamond, hiddenite, moldavite, moonstone, opal, quartz, sapphire, sugilite, topaz, tourmaline, zircon.

Higher teachings: azurite, fluorite, jade, spectrolite, quartz, ruby, sapphire, sugilite, tourmaline.

Hope: amazonite.

House, home: garnet, jade, marble, sard, serpentine.

Illusions, seeing through: amethyst, azurite, chalcedony, pyrite, sodalite.

Ill-wishing, repelling: carnelian, coral, sard.

Improbable situations, handling: spectrolite.

Information: azurite, quartz, sapphire.

Inner guidance: bloodstone, quartz.

Insomnia, treating: agate.

Inspiration: amazonite, amethyst, aquamarine, azurite, garnet, onyx, peridot, pyrite, quartz, sapphire, tourmaline.

Intellect: agate, amber, jade, lapis lazuli, rhodocrosite, serpentine, topaz, tourmaline.

Intolerance: beryl, morganite.

Intuition: amethyst, aquamarine, azurite, citrine, malachite, opal, peridot, quartz, ruby, sapphire, sodalite, topaz, tourmaline.

Invisibility: bloodstone, chrysoprase.

Jealousy: peridot.

Job, career: carnelian, lapis lazuli, scapolite, obsidian.

Justice: amethyst, jade, serpentine.

Karma: calcite, citrine, jade, jet, onyx, quartz, serpentine, shell, tiger's-eye, topaz, obsidian.

Kundalini: amber, bloodstone, garnet.

Lawsuits: see Courts.

Laziness: beryl.

Leadership: iolite, opal, ruby, spinel.

Libraries: sapphire.

Long life: moss agate, beryl, onyx.

Love: aquamarine, aventurine, calcite, coral, emerald, lodestone, malachite, moonstone, rose quartz, ruby, zircon.

Male and female energies: aventurine, tektite, onyx, quartz, sodalite, tiger's-eye.

Marriage: aquamarine, sard.

Medical profession: quartz, spinel, titanite.

Meditation: amethyst, azurite, calcite, coral, emerald, fluorite, geode, jade, malachite, moldavite, quartz, serpentine, shell, sugilite, tanzanite, turquoise, obsidian.

Memory: amethyst, beryl, carnelian, coral, emerald, opal, rhodocrosite, topaz.

Migraines: see Headaches.

Money: agate, amber, bloodstone, calcite, lodestone, malachite, opal, spinel, tourmaline, obsidian, zircon.

Moves: bronzite, jade, serpentine.

Musicians: aventurine, jade, serpentine, tourmaline.

Mystical knowledge: see Higher teachings.

Natural disasters, surviving: spinel.

Nature spirits: moss agate, barite, dioptase, fluorite, holey stones, quartz, staurolite, topaz, tourmaline, wulfenite.

Negative vibrations, shielding against: hematite, jade, serpentine.

New beginnings: agate, emerald, opal, tourmaline.

Nightmares, troubled sleep, removing: chalcedony, garnet, holey stones, jasper, topaz.

Opportunity: garnet.

Overcoming obstacles: agate, hematite.

Past lives: amethyst, coral, fluorite, fossils, garnet, geode, hematite, jasper, malachite, moonstone, opal, petrified wood, quartz, rhodocrosite, shell, staurolite, tiger's-eye, tourmaline, obsidian.

Patience: danburite, spectrolite.

Personal power: agate, cinnabar, jasper, opal, plasma, quartz, ruby.

Physical activity: bronzite, labradorite, obsidian.

Pilots: malachite.

Planning goals: adularia, calcite, hematite, sodalite, topaz, tourmaline.

Plants: dioptase, quartz, tourmaline.

Poverty, reversing: sapphire.

Power: quartz, obsidian.

Pregnancy: dioptase, lapis lazuli, rose quartz.

Privacy: sapphire, jasper.

Prophecy: amethyst, bloodstone, moonstone, opal, quartz, tiger's-eye, topaz, tourmaline, obsidian.

Prosperity: agate, aquamarine, bloodstone, cat's-eye, citrine, crocidolite, emerald, garnet, marble, opal, sapphire, shell, topaz, tourmaline, zircon.

Protection: agate, amethyst, aquamarine, aventurine, beryl, bloodstone, calcite, carnelian, emerald, epidote, garnet, holey stones, jasper, lapis lazuli, pearl, petrified wood, pumice, pyrite, ruby, sapphire, sard, sunstone, tiger's-eye, tourmaline, turquoise, obsidian, zircon.

Psychic abilities: agate, amethyst, apatite, azurite, beryl, crocidolite, heliodor, jet, moonstone, opal, quartz, sapphire, sodalite, spinel, sugilite, tanzanite, tiger's-eye, tourmaline, turquoise, obsidian.

Psychic attack, stopping: smoky quartz, turquoise, obsidian.

Psychic bridge: chrysocolla, quartz, turquoise.

Public speaking: carnelian, emerald. See Communications.

Purification: aquamarine, quartz, tourmaline.

Rain: beryl, turquoise.

Regeneration: alexandrite, garnet, quartz, tourmaline.

Relationships: chrysocolla, pyrite, sapphire.

Releasing: apatite, aventurine, chalcedony, chrysocolla, chrysoprase, jade, moonstone, morganite, petrified wood, quartz, sodalite, tourmaline.

Relieves depression: garnet, jade, jet, lapis lazuli, serpentine, topaz.

Rescue stone: quartz.

Responsibility: aquamarine.

Sacred space: jasper, quartz.

Scrying: agate, beryl, emerald, fluorite, mica, quartz, moonstone, obsidian.

Sea animals, communicating with: lodestone, moldavite.

Seafarers: lodestone, malachite.

Secret enemies, revealing: moonstone.

Security: agate, petrified wood.

Self-confidence: amazonite, aventurine, bloodstone, carnelian, chalcedony, citrine, garnet, iolite, ivory, quartz, rhodonite, sard, spinel, tourmaline.

Self-love: calcite, ivory, quartz.

Severs cording: fire agate, alexandrite, beryl, Boji stones, fluorite, jasper, opal, quartz, zircon.

Sexual attractiveness: opal, sodalite, sunstone, obsidian.

Shaman stone: quartz.

Solving problems: jade, quartz, serpentine.

Soul mates: quartz.

Soul friends: amethyst, quartz.

Speech: see Public speaking.

Speed up manifestation: carnelian, quartz.

Spirit guides, teachers: moss agate, citrine, diopside, lapis lazuli, moonstone, opal, pearl, quartz, spinel, sugilite, topaz, tourmaline, obsidian, zircon.

Spiritual awareness: amethyst, apatite, calcite, emerald, hiddenite, labradorite, lepidolite, moonstone, onyx, pearl, quartz, rhodonite, sphalerite, sugilite, tiger's-eye, vanadinite.

Spiritual mates: quartz.

Stamina: jade, labradorite.

Storms: agate, bloodstone, coral, spinel.

Strategy: fire agate, cassiterite.

Stubbornness: agate, beryl, goshenite, tiger's-eye.

Studying: carnelian, quartz, topaz, tourmaline.

Success: andalusite, sard, obsidian.

Surgery, healing after: bloodstone, hematite.

Survival: chrysocolla, flint, fossils, jade. See Abuse, surviving.

Teachers: quartz, sapphire.

Telepathy: quartz, spinel.

Tension and stress, removing: agate, amethyst, hematite, jade, lapis lazuli, moonstone, peridot, pyrite, quartz, rhodonite, serpentine, obsidian, zircon.

Third eye: moss agate, amethyst, azurite, quartz, sodalite, tiger's-eye.

Time travel: galena, fossils, geode, lodestone, quartz.

Trance: quartz, sapphire, spinel.

Transformation: alexandrite, amethyst, ametrine, azurite, fluorite, garnet, jasper, malachite, onyx, quartz, ruby, shell, tourmaline.

Travel: coral, quartz.

Truth: agate, calcite, chrysoprase, emerald, galena, geode, pearl, pyrite, quartz, sapphire, tiger's-eye, topaz.

Unwanted situations, handling: iolite, malachite.

Useless sacrifices, stopping: quartz.

Victory: agate, chrysoprase, diamond, jet.

Visionary: adularia, agate, amethyst, holey stones, malachite, quartz.

Visualization: aventurine, quartz.

Vitality: moss agate.

Water elementals: agate, aquamarine, fossils, quartz, shell.

Will power: hematite, pyrite.

Writers: amethyst, aventurine, garnet, sapphire, spinel, tourmaline.

Yin/yang: see Male and female energies.

NOTES

Part I. Gate of Stone

The Magical Allure of Stones:

1 *Gems, Crystals and Minerals*, Anna Sofianides and George Harlow.

2 *Cosmic Crystals*, Ra Bonewitz.

Part II. Stones and Their Powers

A Few Facts

1 *The Curious Lore of Precious Stones*, George F. Kunz.

List of Stones A to Z

2 This is found in Pliny's *Natural History*. He gave one of its names as *lyncurius*.

3 *The Magic and Science of Jewels, Vol. 1*, Isidore Kozminsky.

4 *The World of Jewel Stones*, Michael Weinstein.

5 *Gem Magic*, Cornelia Parkinson; *Amber*, Patty Rice.

6 *Gemstones of North America*, John Sinkankas.

7 *The Magic and Science of Jewels, Vol. I.*, Isidore Kozminsky.

8 *A Book of Precious Stones*, Julius Wodiska.

9 *The Occult and Curative Powers of Precious Stones*, William T. Fernie.

10 *The Curious Lore of Precious Stones*, George F. Kunz.

11 Karen and Jerry Gillespie.

12 *Gems: Facts, Fantasies, Superstitions, Legends*, Max Stern.

13 *Gemstones of the World*, Walter Schumann.

14 *Healing Stoned*, Julia Lorusso and Joel Glick.

15 *The Studio Handbook of Minerals*, Hellmuth Boegel.

16 *A Book of Precious Stones*, Julius Wodiska.

17 *A Dictionary of Symbols*, J. E. Cirlot.

18 *Gems*, Robert Webster.

19 *The Magic of Precious Stones*, Mellie Uyldert.

20 *The Occult and Curative Powers of Precious Stones*, William T. Fernie.

21 *The Curious Lore of Precious Stones*, George F. Kunz.

22 *The Studio Handbook of Minerals*, Hellmuth Boegel.

23 Barbara Walker uses these terms to mean garnets. However, any reader will discover that her book *The Book of Sacred Stones: Fact and Fallacy in the Crystal World* spends quite a bit of time disparaging the idea that magic works at all, rather than presenting helpful ways to use stones. I do not recommend this book, except as a source of physical gem facts.

24 *Color Encyclopedia of Gemstones*, Joel E. Arem.

25 *An Introduction to the World's Gemstones*, E. H. Rutland.

26 *Erotic Art of the East*, Philip Rawson.

27 *The World of Jewel Stones*, Michael Weinstein.

28 *Gems*, Robert Webster.

29 *Gems*, Robert Webster.

30 *Legends of Gems*, Horace L. Thomson.

31 Ibid.

32 *The Occult and Curative Powers of Precious Stones*, William T. Fernie.

33 *The Gem Kingdom*, Paul E. Desautels.

34 *The Magic of Minerals*, Olaf Medenbach and Harry Wilk.

35 *Woman's Mysteries*, M. Esther Harding.

36 *Gemstones of North America*, John Sinkankas.

37 *Gemstones of the World*, Walter Schumann.

38 *Michael's Gemstone Dictionary*, Judithann David and J. P. Van Hulle.

39 *A Book of Precious Stones*, Julius Wodiska.

40 *Gems*, Robert Webster.

41 *Legends of Gems*, Horace L. Thomson.

42 *An Introduction to the World's Gemstones*, E. H. Rutland.

43 *The Occult and Curative Powers of Precious Stones*, William T. Fernie.

44 *Magic, Supernaturalism and Religion*, Kurt Seligmann.

45 *Gemstones*, G. F. Herbert Smith.

46 *The Occult and Curative Powers of Precious Stones*, William T. Fernie.

47 *Dictionary of Mythology, Folklore and Symbols*, Gertrude Jobes.

48 *Cunningham's Encyclopedia of Crystal, Gem and Metal Magic.*

49 Marcel Vogel was a noted crystal worker who discovered that cutting crystal increased its storage capacity.

50 *The Magic of Minerals*, Olaf Medenbach and Harry Wilk.

51 *The World of Jewel Stones*, Michael Weinstein.

52 *Gems*, Max Stern and Company.

53 *The Occult and Curative Power of Precious Stones*, William T. Fernie.

54 *Michael's Gemstone Dictionary*, Judithann David and J. P. Van Hulle.

55 *Gypsy Sorcery and Fortune Telling*, Charles Godfrey Leland.

56 *Greek Myths*, Robert Graves.

57 *Pedigree*, Stephen Potter and Laurens Sargent.

58 *Color Encyclopedia of Gemstones*, Joel Arem.

59 *Gems*, Max Stern and Company.

60 *Color Encyclopedia of Gemstones*, Joel Arem.

61 *Gems*, Robert Webster.

62 *Dictionary of Mythology, Folklore and Symbols*, Gertrude Jobes.

63 *Gemstones of North America*, John Sinkankas.

64 The Kalpa Tree was said to be a great mass of glowing gemstones. It had a trunk of diamonds, cat's-eyes, and topaz; roots of sapphire; foliage of zircon and coral; and fruits of pearls, emeralds, and rubies.

Part III. Other Uses for Stone Magic

Practical Spell-Magic with Stones:

1 The Sanskrit names for each chakra is given after the Western one.

Scrying with Stones and Stone Mirrors:

2 *The Mystical Lore of Stones*, George F. Kunz.

BIBLIOGRAPHY

_____. *The Audubon Society Field Guide to North American Rocks and Minerals.* NY: Alfred A. Knopf, 1978.

Aima. *Perfume, Oils, Candles, Seals and Incense.* Foibles Publications, 1971.

Anderson, Frank J. *Riches of the Earth: Ornamental, Precious and Semiprecious Stones.* NY: Windward, 1981.

Arem, Joel E. *Color Encyclopedia of Gemstones.* NY: Van Nostrand Reinhold, 1977.

Axon, Gordon V. *The Wonderful World of Gems.* NY: Criterion Books, 1967.

Baer, Randall N. and Vicki V. *Windows of Light: Quartz Crystals and Self-Transformation.* NY: Harper and Row, 1984.

_____. *The Crystal Connection: A Guidebook for Personal and Planetary Ascension.* NY: Harper and Row, 1987.

Bancroft, Peter. *The World's Finest Minerals and Crystals.* NY: Viking, 1973.

Barrett, Francis. *The Magus.* Secaucus, NJ: Citadel Press, 1980.

Bauer, Jaroslav. *A Field Guide in Color to Minerals, Rocks and Precious Stones.* UK: Octopus Books, 1974.

Bell, Pat and Wright, David. *Rocks and Minerals.* NY: Macmillan, 1985.

Bhattacharya, A. K. *Gem Therapy.* Calcutta, India: Firma KLM Private Ltd., 1992.

Boegel, Hellmuth. *The Studio Handbook of Minerals.* NY: Viking, 1972.

Bonewitz, Ra. *Cosmic Crystals.* San Bernardino, CA: The Borgo Press, 1987.

Bowman, Catherine. *Crystal Awareness.* St. Paul, MN: Llewellyn Publications, 1996.

Bryant, Page. *The Magic of Minerals.* Santa Fe, NM: Sun Publishing, 1987.

Budge, E. A. Wallis. *Amulets and Superstitions.* NY: Dover Publications, 1978. Originally published 1930.

Burbutis, Phillip W. *Quartz Crystals for Healing and Meditation.* Tucson, AZ: Universarium Foundation, 1983.

Camp, John. *Magic, Myth and Medicine.* NY: Taplinger, 1974.

Cayce, Edgar. *Gems and Stones.* Virginia Beach, VA: A.R.E. Press, 1960.

Chocron, Daya Sarai. *Healing With Crystals and Gemstones.* York Beach, MA: Samuel Weiser, 1986.

Cipriani, Nicola. *The Encyclopedia of Rocks and Minerals.* NY: Barnes and Noble, 1996.

Cirlot, J. E. *A Dictionary of Symbols.* NY: Philosophical Library, 1962.

Clark, Andrew. *Rocks and Minerals.* NY: Exeter Books, 1984.

Conway, D. J. *Celtic Magic.* St. Paul, MN: Llewellyn, 1990.

Court, Arthur and Campbell, Ian. *Minerals: Nature's Fabulous Jewels.* NY: Harry N. Abrams, 1974.

Cunningham, Scott. *Cunningham's Encyclopedia of Crystal, Gem and Metal Magic.* St. Paul, MN: Llewellyn Publications, 1990.

_____ and Harrington, David. *Spell Crafts: Creating Magical Objects.* St. Paul, MN: Llewellyn, 1993.

Dake, H. C.; Fleener, Frank L.; and Wilson, Ben Hur. *Quartz Family Minerals.* NY: McGraw-Hill, 1938.

David, Judithann H. and Van Hulle, J. P. *Michael's Gemstone Dictionary.* Orinda, CA: Affinity Press, 1990.

Deeson, A. F. L. *The Collector's Encyclopedia of Rocks and Minerals.* NY: Clarkson N. Potter, 1973.

Desautels, Paul E. *The Mineral Kingdom*. NY: Grosset and Dunlap, 1968.

_____. *Rocks and Minerals*. NY: Grosset and Dunlap, 1974.

_____. *The Gem Kingdom*. NY: Random House, no date.

Dolfyn. *Crystal Wisdom: A Beginner's Guide, Vol. I and II*. Novato, CA: Earthspirit, 1987.

Fernie, P. J., M.D. *The Occult and Curative Powers of Precious Stones*. San Francisco, CA: Harper and Row, 1973.

Fisher, P. J. *The Science of Gems*. NY: Scribner's, 1966.

Fuller, Sue. *Pocket's Rocks and Minerals*. UK: Dorling Kindersley, 1995.

Gait, Robert I. *Exploring Minerals and Crystals*. Toronto: McGraw-Hill Ryerson, 1972.

Galde, Phyllis. *Crystal Healing*. St. Paul, MN: Llewellyn Publications, 1991.

_____ and Bryant, Alice. *The Message of the Crystal Skull: From Atlantis to the New Age*. St. Paul, MN: Llewellyn Publications, 1989.

Gardner, Joy. *Color and Crystals*. Freedom, CA: The Crossing Press, 1988.

Gifford, Edward S., Jr. *The Evil Eye*. NY: Macmillan, 1958.

Gonzalez-Wippler, Migene. *The Complete Book of Amulets and Talismans*. St. Paul, MN: Llewellyn Publications, 1991.

Graves, Robert. *Greek Myths*. UK: Penguin, 1981.

Griffon, T. Wynne. *History of the Occult*. Mallard Press, 1991.

Hall, Callie. *Gem Stones*. NY: DK Publishing, 1994.

Hall, James. *Dictionary of Subjects and Symbols in Art*. Boston, MA: Beacon Press, 1955.

Harding, M. Esther. *Woman's Mysteries: Ancient and Modern*. Boston, MA: Shambhala, 1990.

Harford, Virginia and Milewski, John V. *The Crystal Sourcebook: From Science to Metaphysics*. Santa Fe, NM: Mystic Crystal Publications, 1987.

Harold, Edmund. *Focus on Crystals*. NY: Ballantine Books, 1987.

Hay, John. *Kernels of Energy, Bones of Earth: The Rock in Chinese Art*. NY: China House Gallery, 1985.

Hodges, Doris M. *Healing Stones*. Perry, IO: Pyramid Publishers of Iowa, 1985.

Iorusso, Julia and Glick, Joel. *Healing Stoned: The Therapeutic Use of Gems and Minerals*. Albuquerque, NM: Brotherhood of Life, 1985.

Isaacs, Thelma. *Gemstone and Crystal Energies*. Black Mountain, NC: Lorien House, 1989.

Jobes, Gertrude. *Dictionary of Mythology, Folklore and Symbols*. 3 vols. NY: Scarecrow Press, 1962.

Jones, Wendy and Barry. *The Magic of Crystals*. Australia: Harper Collins, 1996.

Keyte, Geoffrey. *The Healing Crystal*. UK: Blandford, 1989.

Koch, Rudolf. *The Book of Signs*. NY: Dover, 1955.

Kozminsky, Isidore. *The Magic and Science of Jewels and Stones*. Vol. 1 and 2. San Rafael, CA: Cassandra Press, 1988.

Kunz, George Frederick. *The Curious Lore of Precious Stones*. NY: Dover Publications, 1971. Originally printed 1913.

_____. *The Mystical Lore of Precious Stones*. N. Hollywood, CA: Newcastle Publishing, 1986.

_____. *Rings For the Finger*. NY: Dover Publications, 1973. Originally published 1917.

Leek, Sybil. *The Sybil Leek Book of Fortune Telling*. NY: Collier-Macmillan, 1969.

Leland, Charles Godfrey. *Gypsy Sorcery and Fortune Telling.* NY: University Books, 1962.

Lorusso, Julia and Glick, Joel. *Healing Stoned: The Therapeutic Use of Gems and Minerals.* Albuquerque, NM: Brotherhood of Life, 1985.

Lucas, Randolph, ed. *The Illustrated Encyclopedia of Minerals and Rocks.* UK: Octopus Books, 1977.

Lyman, Kennie, ed. *Simon and Schuster's Guide to Gems and Precious Stones.* NY: Simon and Schuster, 1986.

Markham, Ursula. *Fortune-Telling by Crystals and Semi Precious Stones.* UK: Aquarian Press, 1987.

Mendenbach, Olaf and Wilk, Harry. *The Magic of Minerals.* Berlin: Springer-Verlag, 1985.

Metz, Rudolph. *Precious Stones and Other Crystals.* NY: Viking, 1965.

Nassau, Kurt. *Gems Made by Man.* Radnor, PA: Chilton, 1980.

———. *Gemstone Enhancement.* UK: Butterworth's, 1984.

O'Donoghue, Michael. *A Guide to Man-Made Gemstones.* NY: Van Nostrand Reinhold, 1983.

———. *Quartz.* UK: Butterworth's, 1987.

———, ed. *The Encyclopedia of Minerals and Gemstones.* NY: Crescent Books, 1983.

Page, Michael and Ingpen, Robert. *Encyclopedia of Things That Never Were.* NY: Viking Penguin, 1987.

Parkinson, Cornelia M. *Gem Magic.* NY: Fawcett Columbine, 1988.

Paulsen, Kathryn. *The Complete Book of Magic and Witchcraft.* NY: New American Library, 1970.

Pickering, David. *Cassell Dictionary of Superstitions.* UK: Cassell, 1995.

Pollack, Rachel. *Teach Yourself Fortune Telling.* NY: Henry Hold and Co., 1986.

Potter, Carole. *Knock on Wood and Other Superstitions.* NY: Bonanza Books, 1983.

Potter, Stephen and Sargent, Laurens. *Pedigree.* NY: Taplinger, 1974.

Raphaell, Katrina. *Crystal Enlightenment: The Transforming Properties of Crystals and Healing Stones.* Santa Fe, NM: Aurora Press, 1985.

Ravenwolf, Silver. *To Ride a Silver Broomstick.* St. Paul, MN: Llewellyn, 1993.

Rawson, Philip. *Erotic Art of the East.* NY: Putnam, 1968.

Rea, John D. *Patterns of the Whole: Vol. 1, Healing and Quartz Crystals.* Boulder, CO: Two Trees Publishing, 1986.

Renee, Janina. *Tarot Spells.* St. Paul, MN: Llewellyn, 1990.

Rice, Patty C. *Amber: The Golden Gem of the Ages.* NY: Van Nostrand Reinhold, 1980.

Richardson, Wally and Huett, Lenora. *Spiritual Value of Gem Stones.* Marina del Rey, CA: DeVorss and Co., 1980.

Rose, Donna. *Love Spells.* Hialeah, FL: Mi-World, no date.

———. *Magic of Astrology.* Hialeah, FL: Mi-World, 1978.

———. *Money Spells.* Hialeah, FL: Mi-World, 1978.

Rouse, John D. *Garnet.* UK: Butterworth's, 1986.

Rutland, E. H. *An Introduction to the World's Gemstones.* NY: Doubleday, 1974.

Sanborn, William B. *Oddities of the Mineral World.* NY: Van Nostrand Reinhold, 1976.

Schumann, Walter. *Gemstones of the World.* NY: Sterling, 1977.

Seligmann, Kurt. *Magic, Supernaturalism and Religion.* NY: Pantheon, 1948.

Showers, Paul. *Fortune Telling For Fun and Profit.* NY: Bell Publishing, 1985.

Silbey, Uma. *The Complete Crystal Guidebook.* NY: Bantam Books, 1987.

Sinkankas, John. *Gemstones of North America.* Princeton, NJ: D. Van Nostrand, 1959.

Skelton, Robin. *Talismanic Magic.* York Beach, ME: Samuel Weiser, 1985.

Smith, G. F. Herbert. *Gemstones.* NY: Pitman, 1958.

Smith, Michael G. *Crystal Power.* St. Paul, MN: Llewellyn Publications, 1985.

————. *Crystal Spirit.* St. Paul, MN: Llewellyn, 1990.

————. *Crystal Warrior: Shamanic Transformation and Projection of Universal Energy.* St. Paul, MN: Llewellyn Publications, 1993.

Sofianides, Anna S.; Harlow, George E.; et al. *Gems, Crystals and Minerals.* NY: Simon and Schuster, 1990.

Spencer, L. J. *A Key to Precious Stones.* NY: Emerson Books, 1959.

Stafford, Penny. *Healing Stones.* Minneapolis, MN: self-published, no date.

Stein, Diane. *The Women's Book of Healing.* St. Paul, MN: Llewellyn, 1993.

————. *The Women's Spirituality Book.* St. Paul, MN: Llewellyn, 1987.

Stern, Max and Company. *Gems: Facts, Fantasies, Superstitions, Legends.* NY: Max Stern and Co., 1946.

Sullivan, Kevin. *The Crystal Handbook.* NY: Signet, 1987.

Thomas, William and Pavitt, Kate. *The Book of Talismans, Amulets and Zodiacal Gems.* N. Hollywood, CA: Wilshire Book Co., 1970.

Thompson, C. J. S. *The Mysteries and Secrets of Magic.* NY: Barnes and Noble, 1993.

Thomson, Horace L. *Legends of Gems.* Los Angeles, CA: Graphic Press, 1937.

Trachtenberg, Joshua. *Jewish Magic and Superstition: A Study in Folk Religion.* NY: Atheneum, 1984.

Troyer, Patricia. *Crystal Personalities: A Quick Reference to Special Forms of Crystal.* Peoria, AZ: Stone People Publishing Co., 1995.

Trussell, Daniel. *Mineral Attunements For Healing and Development.* Atlanta, GA: Browning Press, 1987.

Uyldert, Mellie. *The Magic of Precious Stones.* UK: Turnstone Press, 1981.

Wade, Frank B. *A Text-Book of Precious Stones.* NY: Putnam's, 1918.

Walker, Barbara G. *The Book of Sacred Stones.* San Francisco, CA: HarperCollins, 1989.

————. *The Woman's Dictionary of Symbols and Sacred Objects.* San Francisco, CA: Harper and Row, 1988.

Webster, Robert. *Gems: Their Sources, Descriptions and Identification.* UK: Butterworth's, 1983.

Weinstein, Michael. *The World of Jewel Stones.* NY: Sheridan House, 1958.

Whitlock, Herbert P. *The Story of the Gems.* NY: Emerson Books, 1963.

Wodiska, Julius. *A Book of Precious Stones.* NY: Putnam's, 1909.

Woolley, Alan, ed. *The Illustrated Encyclopedia of the Mineral Kingdom.* NY: Larousse, 1978.

Zim, Herbert S. and Shaffer, Paul R. *Rocks and Minerals: A Guide to Familiar Minerals, Gems, Ores and Rocks.* NY: Golden Press, 1957.

INDEX

BOOKS BY THE CROSSING PRESS

Laying on of Stones

By D.J. Conway

Stones can be used to protect and heal you, your family, and your home, but where to place them is often a source of difficulty. Probably the most important question frequently asked is where to place them on your body. D. J. Conway has supplied you with forty detailed diagrams, showing you exactly how to place a variety of stones to help your body heal itself of illness or enrich your life through a magical manifestation of desires.

$10.95 • Paper • ISBN 1-58091-029-7

The Little Book of Candle Magic

By D.J. Conway

This little, but informative, book offers the historical purpose of candles and fire in rituals as well as instruction on the use of color, incense, herbs, stones, and spells to bring abundance and well-being into your life.

Pocket Guide to Crystals & Gemstones

By Sirona Knight

This book describes crystals and gemstones and tells you where they can be found, what are their corresponding energy fields, how they should be chosen, and how they are cleaned and used.

$6.95 • Paper • ISBN 0-89594-947-4

Healing with Flower and Gemstone Essences

By Diane Stein

Instructions for choosing and using flowers and gems are combined with descriptions of their effect on emotional balance. Includes instructions for making flower essences and for matching essences to hara line chakras for maximum benefit.

$14.95 • Paper • ISBN 0-89594-856-7

Healing with Gemstones and Crystals

By Diane Stein

More than 200 gemstones and their healing properties are listed. Details on how to choose and use the Earth's precious gems are supplemented by explanations of the significance of this type of healing.

$14.95 • Paper • ISBN 0-89594-831-1

To receive a current catalog from The Crossing Press
please call toll-free, 800-777-1048.
www.crossingpress.com